Cooking for Diabetics

Diet plays a very important role in any disease, more so in diabetes.

By

Satarupa Banerjee

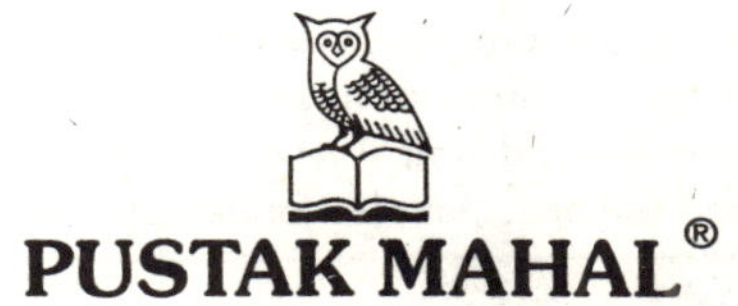

PUSTAK MAHAL®

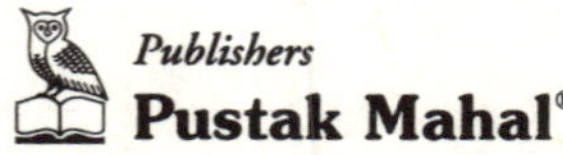

Publishers
Pustak Mahal®

Administrative office and sale centre
J-3/16 , Daryaganj, New Delhi-110002
☎ 23276539, 23272783, 23272784 • *Fax:* 011-23260518
E-mail: info@pustakmahal.com • *Website:* www.pustakmahal.com

Branches
Bengaluru: ☎ 080-22234025 • *Telefax:* 080-22240209
E-mail: pustak@airtelmail.in • pustak@sancharnet.in
Mumbai: ☎ 022-22010941, 022-22053387
E-mail: rapidex@bom5.vsnl.net.in
Patna: ☎ 0612-3294193 • *Telefax:* 0612-2302719
E-mail: rapidexptn@rediffmail.com

ISBN 978-81-223-0643-9

Edition: 2013

Printed at : Sharma Printers, Delhi.

PREFACE

Diabetic diet has changed over the years and is no longer bland, and tasteless food with heavy restrictions. I have adapted and modified a number of recipes so that they retain the flavour but are cooked according to the dietary needs of a diabetic patient.

Eating is one of the most pleasurable activities of our lives. And a housewife spends the better part of the day preparing meals for the family. Being a working housewife, I quite appreciate how difficult it is to cater to a patient in the family, when you have to cook two sets of meals.

Here is a book that caters to the diabetic with healthy and delicious recipes which the whole family can enjoy. It is also great for people who want to eat light but good food and in general have a healthy diet.

Good health to you all.

—Author

Preface

CONTENTS

INTRODUCTION

There is no disease which provokes greater thought on diet than diabetes.

What is diabetes ? Diabetes mellitus, to give the disease its full name, is a chronic metabolic disorder, with a strong hereditary base, associated with high blood sugar and usually with the passage of sugar in the urine.

Diabetes is caused by an inadequate supply of insulin which is produced by the pancreas to metabolise sugar and starch. There is an excessive accumulation of glucose (a type of sugar) in the blood. Sugar provides us with energy and is an essential part of our diet. Apart from sugar itself, our main source is carbohydrates which is found aplenty in potatoes, bread, rice, cake and biscuits. They are converted during digestion to glucose which is absorbed into the blood stream and carried to energize the muscles and other tissues, or stored in the liver for future use.

Normally the hormone insulin (produced by the pancreatic gland) controls the levels of glucose in our blood, but in diabetes, it fails to do so.

This book is not about the disease itself so I won't go into the details of symptoms etc. But all would agree that a proper diet programme can have a miraculous effect on a diabetic.

Nutrition is a part of life where we are the most vulnerable. It hurts, when we are deprived of our favourite foods, if our meal times are disrupted; when we can't sit down to eat the same food as the rest of the family members.

For a diabetic the right diet is at least half his treatment when he is on insulin. In some cases, it is the whole of it - when he is not on insulin.

Even a few years ago, the diet scene for diabetics was quite gloomy. Thankfully, things have changed now. You can have an almost normal diet.

There are three golden rules for all diabetics who intend to take their diet and diabetic control seriously, whether they need insulin injections or not.

1. Control you intake of calories in order to achieve or stay at your ideal body weight. For most diabetics this will involve a reduction of calories. If you are moderately overweight, you will probably be able to reach your ideal weight by eating low calorie foods and by low calorie recipes given in this book.
2. If you are very overweight you will only be able to achieve this by sticking to a planned daily calorie limit and the calories in all the food and drink you consume. Your doctor or dietician will give you the information you need to do this.
3. Eat regular meals. This is a sensible practice for diabetics and non-diabetics alike. However, balancing insulin with food is essential, if you take insulin and wish to achieve good control regular meals are essential.

Until a few years ago, a diabetic was advised to reduce all carbohydrate foods both starchy (potatoes and rice etc) and sugary. Such diets were quite often high in fat; but now the diabetic patient is asked to take a diet which is high in fibre and carbohydrates and low in fat.

This has quite a few advantages. The reduced amount of fat in its turn helps to lower blood cholesterol levels (which are often raised in people with diabetes) and so hopefully in the long run reduces the risk of heart attacks, to which diabetics are particularly prone. Also, the salt intake should be curtailed for the same reason.

Dietary fibre or roughage helps to lower blood sugar levels. And many diabetics who are overweight need to lose weight. A high fibre diet is filling which helps make slimming easier.

To put it in a nutshell, a diabetic should avoid sugar, root vegetables like yam, colocasia, tapioca etc., fruits like banana, chickoo etc. Rice and potatoes should be taken in moderation. Pulses and legumes play an important part in Indian diet, particularly the vegetarian one, as they supply a fair quantity of protein. But do not serve very thick dals and definitely not with ghee or butter. Sprouted beans are always welcome. Sprouting and fermenting help utilise starchy food better.

One helping of meat, fish, chicken or egg can be taken at each meal for all diabetics taking a mixed diet.

Milk should always be skimmed, that is the fat content removed. Curd or paneer should always be homemade from the skimmed milk. Milk, paneer and curd made from soyabeans are also okay.

Guava, citrus fruits, papaya and leafy vegetables can be eaten. Instead of nuts, eat pumpkin seeds, sesame seeds and poppy seeds.

While following the recipes in this book, remember oil is always unsaturated and salt should be reduced. Even if the recipe states salt to taste use only half amount of what you would normally add, as a low sodium diet is recommended for diabetics.

This book offers a guideline only. It is not possible to weigh each ingredient and count every calorie because a diabetic patient has to follow a diet for the rest of his life. Above all, do consult your physician in case of any doubt and follow his advice.

I hope the recipes in this book will help make the high fibre, low fat diet an enjoyable way of eating. Once you become accustomed to it you'll find that you prefer it to the traditional diet you have been eating before. What's more, very soon your whole family will come to love it as well.

I hope that diabetics will lead the way to healthier eating for the non-diabetics too.

Abbreviations

gm	-	gram
kg	-	kilogram
l	-	litre
ml	-	millilitre
tsp	-	teaspoon
tbsp	-	tablespoon

Weights and Measures

Recipes in this book use the standard measuring set of cups and spoons.

A graduated set of four cups measuring one cup, a half, a third and a quarter cup.

A graduated set of 4 spoons — tablespoon, teaspoon, a half and a quarter spoon.

1 tbsp = 3 tsp 1 cup = 16 tbsp

All measurements are level unless stated otherwise.

Here are a few tips on how to measure.

Liquids: Place the measuring cup on a flat surface and pour the liquid to the required level. The spoons should also be filled to the level.

Dry Ingredients: These should be spooned lightly into the cup until heaped, then levelled off with a straight edged knife or spatula. Never pack the ingredients down or shake or tap the cup. And unless specified, measure before sifting.

Moist Ingredients: It is these ingredients, like shortening and brown sugar, that have to be packed in lightly. Press the fat into the cup so that air spaces are forced out. Level fat to straight edge when full.

Beverages

Masala Tea

Ingredients (Serves 4)

- 2 cups of water
- 2 tea bags
- 150 ml low fat milk
- 5 cm stick of cinnamon
- 1/4 tsp cardamom powder
- 1 tsp peppercorns
- Sugar free sweetener to taste

Preparation

Bring water to a boil in a saucepan and add the teabags. Remove from heat and steep 10 minutes. Discard tea bags. Add the milk, spices and sweetener. Heat and keep covered on low heat for about 10 minutes. Strain and serve.

Tomato Cocktail

Ingredients (Serves 4)

- 8 large, red ripe tomatoes
- 1 small onion
- 2 ribs celery with leaves
- 3 sprigs parsley
- 1/2 cup of water
- 1 bay leaf
- 1/2 tsp salt
- 1/4 tsp pepper
- 1 tsp Worcestershire sauce

Preparation

Quarter the tomatoes. Slice the onion; chop the celery and parsley. Simmer the vegetables with water and the bay leaf for 1/2 an hour or till very soft. Let cool a little and blend. Strain and serve with salt, pepper and Worcestershire sauce. Serve chilled.

Try varying the flavour with other combinations like tomato and orange, tomato and cucumber etc.

Diabetic Pep Up

Ingredients (Serves 4)

- 250 gm jamun
- 1/4 cup bel pulp
- 1/2 tsp salt
- 4 cups of water
- 1/4 tsp freshly ground pepper

Preparation

Wash the jamuns. Take out the seeds and blend the fruit and the bel pulp in a processor. Add all the remaining ingredients. Serve chilled.

This jamun and bel fruit drink is almost like a medicine for a diabetic. All the parts of jamun are used in the treatment of diabetes. The fruits, seeds and leaves all possess curative properties.

Fruity Curd Smoothie

Ingredients (Serves 4)

- 1 cup chopped pineapple
- 1 cup chopped papaya
- 1 cup fresh orange juice
- 4 cups fresh thick curd
- Sugar free sweetener equivalent of 1 tbsp sugar

Preparation

Put all the fruits in a blender. Add the orange juice and sweetener and blend together. Slowly add the curd and keep blending till smooth. Make this smoothie thick or thin as per your taste. Serve chilled in a tall glass.

Don't think cereals are the only option for a quick breakfast every morning. Try this alternative which is fast to cook and healthy to boost.

Soups

Dumpling Soup

Ingredients (Serves 4)

For Soup

- 6 cups chicken stock or vegetable stock
- A handful of fresh coriander

For Dumplings

- 4 tbsp fenugreek leaves, very finely chopped
- 1 cup gramflour
- 1/2 cup atta
- 1/2 tsp oil
- 1 tsp ginger paste
- 1/2 tsp chilli powder
- 1/4 tsp soda bicarb
- Pinch of turmeric
- Pinch of salt

Preparation

Mix all the ingredients for the dumplings into a stiff dough with water. Form into small balls. Put the stock to boil. If using chicken stock, refrigerate for a couple of hours to let the fat congeal. Discard the fat and only then use the stock. Once the stock comes to a boil, add the dumplings gently and cook till they float on top. Serve garnished with coriander leaves. You may add lime juice to taste.

Consomme Julienne

Ingredients (Serves 4)

- 850 ml stock
- 1 medium carrot
- 2 sticks celery
- 1 small onion
- 2 cloves
- 1 egg
- 125 gm minced chicken
- 10 peppercorns
- Salt to taste
- 1 tbsp vinegar

Preparation

Refrigerate the stock overnight. You'll find the fat congealed on top. Remove the fat and discard. Cut the carrot and celery into juliennes, that is matchlike strips. Stick the cloves into the onion. Beat the egg into the stock. Add the vegetables and minced chicken. Put to boil. Add the onion, peppercorn, salt and vinegar when it comes to a boil. Simmer covered for one hour. Strain and serve. Only the soup is drunk; the rest discarded. Garnish with finely chopped parsley.

This healthy soup makes a very good mid morning or evening snack.

Creamy Matar Paneer Soup

Ingredients (Serves 2)

- $2^1/_2$ cups chicken stock
- 1 tbsp refined oil
- 1/4 cup chopped onion
- 1 tsp atta
- 1 cup shelled peas
- 1/4 cup soft paneer
- 2 tsp lime juice
- 2 tbsp chopped green chilli
- Salt to taste
- Freshly ground pepper to taste

Preparation

The stock should be fat-free. To achieve this, refrigerate the stock overnight. The fat will congeal on top. Remove and discard. Heat the oil in a large saucepan. Add the onion and saute till transparent. Add the atta and stir for 1 minute. Stir in the stock. Add the peas, simmer with lid on till the peas are done. Transfer half the mixture to a blender and puree with the paneer till smooth. Add the lime juice. Heat the puree with the remaining soup, chilli, salt and pepper. Serve hot.

The paneer in this soup provides a richness, surprisingly similar to that of cream, but without the fat and cholesterol.

Bathua and Orange Soup

Ingredients (Serves 2)

- 250 gm bathua greens
- 1/2 tsp salt
- 1 tbsp homemade pulpy paneer
- 1/3 cup milk
- 1 cup fresh orange juice
- 1/2 tsp pepper
- Juice of half a lime
- A few lime slices for garnishing

Preparation

Wash the bathua leaves in several changes of water; discarding the tough stems; shred finely. Pressure cook with 1/2 cup of water and salt for 5 minutes. Cool, blend and strain. Blend the paneer and milk together. Heat the soup, orange juice and pepper together. Mix in the paneer. Remove. Serve hot, sprinkled with lime juice and garnished with lime slices.

Green Pea Rasam

Ingredients (Serves 4)

- 2 cups shelled green peas
- 4 tsp coriander seeds
- 1 tsp cumin seeds
- 1/2 tsp peppercorns
- 1 dry red chilli (optional)
- 6 cloves garlic
- 1 tbsp tamarind pulp

Preparation

Cook the shelled green peas in 1 cup of water. Keep aside. Dry roast the coriander, cumin seeds, peppercorns and red chilli if using, together. Grind these alongwith 1/3 of the cooked peas, using the water in which the peas were boiled. Add 4 cups of water to the ground paste and bring to a boil. After 5 minutes, add the remaining peas along with the salt and tamarind pulp. Mix well. You may add more water if you want a thinner rasam.

Variation: Use broccoli florets the same way.

TOMATO RASAM

Ingredients (Serves 4)

- 1 large tomato
- A handful of arhar dal
- 4 cups of water
- 1/2 tsp grated ginger
- Salt to taste
- 1 slit green chilli (optional)
- 1 tbsp fresh coriander, finely chopped
- 4 curry leaves

For tempering

- 1 tsp refined oil
- 1 pinch mustard seeds
- 1 pinch cumin seed
- A small pinch of asafoetida

Preparation

Chop the tomato and pressure cook with the dal, water, ginger and salt for 15 minutes. Blend and strain. Heat the oil in a karahi. Temper with the mustard seeds, cumin and asafoetida. Add the rasam. When it comes to a boil, add the green chilli, if using, fresh coriander and curry leaves. Serve hot.

Salads

Paneer Fruit Salad

Ingredients (Serves 4)

- 4 tbsp grated paneer
- Different types of fruits like orange, pear, apple, grape
- Juice of 1 orange
- Juice of 1 lime
- Cherries for garnishing

Preparation

Peel and dice the pear and apple. Segment the orange. Halve the grapes. Divide the fruits equally between 4 individual dessert bowls. Mix orange juice and lime juice and pour over the fruits. Garnish with grated paneer and cherries.

Paushtik Salad (Nutritious Salad)

Ingredients (Serves 4)

- 1 small radish
- 1 cup sprouted wheat
- 1 cup shredded tender spinach, leaves only
- 50 gm soya paneer, diced

For Dressing

- 3 cloves garlic, minced
- 3 tsp vinegar or lime juice
- Salt and pepper to taste

Preparation

Grate the radish. Combine the salad ingredients in a bowl. Mix the dressing and pour over the salad. Chill and serve.

Variation: Use any other sprout, like moong, chana or moth etc. A judicious combination of nutritious salad ingredients.

Som Tam (Thai Papaya Salad)

Ingredients (Serves 6)

- 1 small raw papaya
- 100 gm French beans or long beans (barbati)
- 2 capsicums
- 2 tomatoes
- 1 or 2 green chillies
- 1/4 cup green coriander
- 1 tbsp lime juice
- 1 tbsp fish sauce (optional)
- 1 tbsp tomato ketchup
- 1 tbsp refined oil
- A pinch of salt

Preparation

Peel and grate the papaya. Blanch beans or 'barbati' and cut into 2 cm pieces. Chop the capsicum, tomato and green chilli. Put the papaya and beans in a bowl and pound roughly with a heavy ladle. Add the capsicum, tomato, green chilli, green coriander, lime juice, fish sauce (if using), ketchup, oil and salt. Toss well to coat all ingredients evenly before serving.

Glass Noodles Salad

Ingredients (Serves 2)

- 1/2 packet glass noodles
- 200 gm minced chicken
- 2 tbsp refined oil
- 100 gm shrimps
- 2 tbsp vinegar
- 2 tomatoes
- 2 capsicums
- 1 tbsp soyabean sauce
- 1 tbsp fish sauce (optional)
- 1 tbsp tomato ketchup
- 1 tbsp lime juice
- 1 tbsp vinegar
- 2 green chillies
- Salt and pepper to taste

Preparation

Boil water in a saucepan that will hold the noodles comfortably. Remove from heat and soak the glass noodles in it for half an hour. Shell, devein, wash and cook the shrimps till just done. Blanch, deseed and cut tomatoes into juliennes. Discard the seeds and cut capsicums into juliennes, too, chop the green chillies. Heat the oil in a pan. Add the mince and stir well. Cover and cook till done. Drain the noodles and mix with the chicken. Add the cooked shrimp and the rest of the ingredients. Toss to mix well. Keep aside for 10 minutes and serve.

Fenugreek Sprout Salad

Ingredients (Serves 2)

- 1 small capsicum
- 1 large tomato
- 1 small onion
- 1/3 cup fenugreek sprouts
- 1 cup whole Bengal gram sprouts
- Few lettuce leaves

For Dressing:

- 1 tbsp lime juice
- 1 tsp green capsico sauce
- Salt and pepper to taste

Preparation

Wash, deseed and cut capsicum into juliennes. Cut tomato into bite size pieces. Slice the onion. Combine all the salad ingredients. Mix the dressing ingredients together and pour over the salad. Mix well. Serve chilled over crisp lettuce leaves.

Variation: Use a combination of different coloured capsicums for a better visual effect.

Fenugreek is mostly used in its seed form and is found more often in pickles than curries. It is bitter, pungent, and a good rejuvenator. Here the seeds are used in a sprouted form.

Mixed Sprout Salad

Ingredients (Serves 4)

- 1/4 cup moth sprouts
- 1/4 cup whole green gram sprouts
- 1/4 cup black eyed beans sprouts
- 1 small carrot
- 1 small radish
- 2 medium onions, finely sliced
- 100 gm fresh pomegranate seeds

For Dressing

- 1 green chilli, finely chopped
- 2.5 cm piece of ginger, grated
- 2 tsp lime juice
- Pinch of salt and pepper to taste

Preparation

For sprouting any seed, choose good quality seeds. Clean and discard any diseased seeds. Wash thoroughly and soak in cold water for 10-12 hours. Drain well. Tie the seeds in a fine muslin cloth and hang the bundle in a warm place. Keep sprinkling some water, morning and evening. Sprouting will start within 6-7 hours. For longer sprouts, allow them to grow for at least 3-4 days. Peel and grate the carrot and radish. Add sliced onion with sprouts and pomegranate seeds. Mix the dressing ingredients together and pour over the salad. Toss so that the dressing coats the ingredients well. Chill and serve.

Variation: This also makes a good sandwich filling.

Sprouts are a store house of energy. So, try to include it in a diabetic diet as often as you can.

Bengal Gram Raita

Ingredients (Serves 6)

- 2 cups roasted Bengal gram
- 2 cups fresh curd
- 1/2 tsp salt
- 1/2 tsp pepper
- 1/2 tsp roasted and powdered cumin seeds
- 1/2 tsp black salt
- 1 tbsp chopped fresh coriander
- 1 green chilli, chopped

Preparation

Roasted chana generally comes with the husk. Remove the husk and soak in lukewarm water for half an hour. The curd should, preferably, be homemade using fat free milk. Whisk the curd till smooth and add all spices. Lastly, drain the chick peas and add to the curd. Garnish with the coriander and green chilli.

Roasted Bengal gram has a beneficial effect on diabetics. Its consumption results in considerable reduction in blood sugar levels, improves glucose tolerance and general condition.

Fruit Raita

Ingredients (Serves 6)

- 1/2 kg curd
- 1 tomato
- 1 small onion
- 1 small cucumber
- 1/2 small green capsicum
- 1/2 small red capsicum
- 1 small apple
- 1 pear
- 1 guava
- A pinch of chaat masala
- 1/2 tsp black salt
- A handful of fresh coriander

Preparation

Hang the curd tied in a muslin for half an hour, till part of the whey drains off. Cut all the vegetables and fruits into tiny pieces. Mix all together and add the chaat masala and salt. Garnish with coriander leaves. Chill and serve.

Cheese Dip

Ingredients (Serves 6)

- 250 gm homemade pulpy paneer
- 1/2 tsp garlic paste
- 150 gm hung curd
- 1 green chilli finely chopped

Preparation

Blend the paneer till smooth. Add garlic paste and curd and blend again. Add green chilli and put in a serving bowl. Chill for 2 hours.

Serve with vegetable crudites—which means different vegetables like carrot, capsicum, cucumber, celery cut in finger-sized pieces. Can be served as toppings of canapes, too.

Bread Mayonnaise

Ingredients (Makes 1 cup)

- 3/4 cup fresh curd
- 2 slices bread
- 1/2 tsp salt
- Pinch of sugar
- 1/2 tsp mustard powder
- 1/4 tsp pepper powder
- 2 tsp refined oil

Preparation

Put the curd in a strainer and press lightly to drain some of the whey. Trim the crusts of the bread slices. Crumble the bread and soak in the curd. Put in the blender along with the seasonings and oil. Blend till smooth and has a ketchup-like consistency.

Regular mayonnaise uses too much oil making it a taboo for the diabetics. Prepare the above recipe instead, which has hardly any oil, without the taste suffering.

MAIN DISH–VEGETARIAN

SHUKTO

(VEGETABLE MEDLEY WITH NEEM LEAVES)

Ingredients (Serves 3-4)

- 1 1/2 tsp paanch phoran, powdered
- 1 tbsp mustard oil
- Handful of tender neem leaves
- 250 gm raw papaya
- 1 tbsp poppy seeds
- 2.5 cm piece of ginger
- 2 tsp mustard seeds
- 1 tsp salt

Preparation

Heat 1 tsp of the oil in a small pan and stir fry the neem leaves and set aside. Wash, peel and cut the papaya in small cubes. Grind the mustard seeds, poppy seeds and ginger. Heat the remaining oil in a karahi and season with the rest of the paanch phoran. When they pop, add the papaya pieces and saute 2 minutes. Add the ground spice, salt and saute another minute. Add enough water to cook the papaya and neem leaves and cover. This has a soupy gravy so add water accordingly. Remove when done. Sprinkle the paanch phoran on top and serve at room temperature with boiled rice at the very beginning of the meal.

Variation: Instead of papaya, lauki, ash gourd or ripe cucumber (deseeded) can be used as well.

Shukto is a popular Bengali dish; served at the very beginning of the meal. It works as an appetiser. The vegetables can be varied, but a bitter ingredient is a must. Here I have used neem leaves. *They are extremely rich in vitamin A, B and C, iron, calcium, phosphorus, copper, potassium, magnesium, sulphur and chlorine. Such a rich combination of nutrients gives them a great cleansing effect. Like the bitter gourd, its effect is most beneficial on the diabetics.*

Dal Stuffed Bitter Gourd

Ingredients (Serves 5)

- 10 medium bitter gourds
- 70 gm masoor dal
- 70 gm moong dal
- 70 gm arhar dal
- Refined oil as needed
- 1 tomato, chopped
- Juice of 1 lime
- Salt to taste

Grind together:

- 1 medium onion
- 1 green chilli
- 1/2 tsp turmeric powder
- 1/2 tsp coriander seeds, roasted
- 3 cloves garlic

Preparation

Wash the bitter gourds. Make a slit in the middle lengthwise and take out the seeds and pith. Steam the gourds till half done. Reserve. Cook all the dals in a little water till soft. Drain and keep aside. Heat 1 tsp oil in a non-stick pan. Add the ground paste. Add the cooked dals and salt; stir-fry. Add the chopped tomato and fry the dal mix till the tomato gets well-mixed. Add lime juice and keep aside. Divide the dal mixture in 10 equal portions. Stuff into the prepared bitter gourds. Don't stuff very tightly or it will spill while frying. Heat 1 tbsp oil in a non-stick skillet and fry the stuffed gourds till a light brown.

Bitter gourd contains a hypoglycemic or insulin like property, also known as plant insulin which is highly beneficial in lowering blood and urine sugar level.

Broken Wheat Khichdi

Ingredients (Serves 4)

- 1 cup mixed vegetables
- 200 gm dalia or broken wheat
- 1 coconut, grated
- 1 tbsp refined oil
- 50 gm Bengal gram dal
- 3 cloves
- 2 green cardamoms
- Pinch of nutmeg powder
- 1 tsp salt
- 3 tbsp chopped fresh coriander
- 1 tbsp groundnuts (optional)

Preparation

By mixed vegetables I mean cauliflower, beans and peas. Clean and wash dalia. Extract 1 cup thick milk from the coconut. Reserve. Roast the dalia in a pan for 5 minutes. Cool. Heat the oil and fry the gram dal for 2 minutes. Add the vegetables and saute for a minute. Add 2 cups of water and bring to a boil. Add the spices, salt and dalia and stir well. Cook on a low heat till the water gets absorbed. Add the coconut milk and continue cooking till done. Garnish with groundnuts, if using and fresh coriander.

Sauteed Amaranth

Ingredients (Serves 4)

- 2 cups amaranth, chopped
- 1 green chilli, slit
- 1 tsp refined oil
- 1 small onion, finely chopped
- Salt to taste

Preparation

Wash the amaranth in several changes of water and then chop. Do not wash afterwards. Heat the oil in a karahi. Add the onion and stir fry till soft. Add the amaranth, slit green chilli and salt. The amaranth will release its own water. Cook uncovered, stirring continually, till the water dries up. It helps if you use a non-stick pan.

Variation: Use any other green leafy vegetable like spinach, bathua etc.

Leafy vegetables are highly recommended for a diabetic diet. Amaranth is rich in vitamin A. Also prevents deficiency of vitamins B_1, B_2 and C, calcium, iron and potassium.

Brinjal Caviar

Ingredients (Serves 4)

- 1 large brinjal
- 1 onion finely chopped
- 6 cloves of garlic
- 1/2 cup hung curd
- 1/2 cup pulpy paneer
- Salt and pepper to taste

Preparation

Smear the brinjal with a little oil and roast over flame till baked and soft; peel. Grind the onion and garlic in a mixie. Add the curd and paneer and blend till smooth. Finally add the brinjal, salt and pepper and blend till well mixed. Can be served cold on toasted bread or as it is with chappatis.

Fenugreek Seeds Curry

Ingredients (Serves 4)

- 1/2 cup fenugreek seeds
- 1 tsp refined oil
- 1/2 tsp cumin seeds
- Pinch of asafoetida
- 1/2 tsp chilli powder
- 1/2 tsp turmeric powder
- 1 tbsp coriander powder
- 2 tsp lime juice
- A handful of chopped fresh coriander
- 1 tsp salt

Preparation

Wash and soak fenugreek seeds in $1^1/_2$ cups of water for 3-4 hours. Boil in the same water till tender and the water absorbed. Heat the oil in a non-stick skillet. Season with cumin seeds; when it stops spluttering, add asafoetida. Mix the chilli, turmeric, and coriander powders in 4 tbsp water and add to the pan. Stir fry over medium heat till the mixture dries up. Add the boiled fenugreek seeds and 1/2 cup of water. Bring to a boil; simmer 2 minutes. Remove from heat; sprinkle lime juice and garnish with coriander leaves.

It has been medically proved that fenugreek seeds diminish reactive hyperglycemia in diabetic patients. Consumption of this seed also significantly lowers the levels of glucose, serum cholesterol and tryglycerides of diabetic patients.

Stuffed Brinjal Bake

Ingredients (Serves 4)

- 4 medium brinjals
- 1/2 tsp salt

For Stuffing

- 200 gm soyabean granules
- 1 tbsp refined oil
- 2 medium onions, chopped
- 100 gm mushrooms
- 4 tbsp brown breadcrumbs
- 4 tbsp chopped parsley or fresh coriander
- 1/2 tsp ground mace
- Salt and pepper to taste

For Tomato Sauce

- 1 tbsp refined oil
- 1 onion, finely chopped
- 5 tbsp tomato puree
- Pinch of ajwain
- Pinch of pepper

Preparation

Cut the brinjals in halves lengthways and scoop out the flesh, leaving a 5 mm shell, sprinkle the shells and flesh with salt and leave for half an hour; rinse throughly and pat dry. Chop the flesh.

Stuffing: Soak the soyabean granules in boiling water for half an hour. Strain and squeeze dry. Heat the oil. Add the onion and fry gently for 5 minutes until transparent. Add the brinjal flesh and mushrooms and continue to cook for a further 5 minutes, stirring continually. Remove from heat and add the soya granules. Mix well. Mix the breadcrumbs, parsley or coriander, mace, salt and pepper.

Tomato Sauce: Heat the oil in a saucepan and fry the onions gently until transparent. Add the puree and cook for a few minutes. Stir in the crushed ajwain and a cup of water; cover and simmer for 25-30 minutes. Taste and add pepper. Place the brinjal shells in a baking dish and spoon in the stuffing. Pour the tomato sauce over and around the shells and bake for 25-30 minutes at a temperature of 190° C/380° F.

Ratatouille

Ingredients (Serves 4)

- 4 large tomatoes
- 1 onion
- 1 brinjal
- 100 gm tinda
- 100 gm snake gourd
- 100 gm bottle gourd
- 1 tsp salt
- 1 tsp pepper powder
- Pinch of ajwain, crushed
- 1/2 cup vegetable stock

Preparation

Chop the tomatoes and slice the rest of the vegetables. Place the onion, brinjal, tinda, snake gourd and bottle gourd in an ovenproof dish. Add the salt, pepper and ajwain to the vegetable stock and mix well. Arrange the tomatoes over the vegetables and pour in the stock. Bake in an oven preheated to 190°C/ 380° F for 30 - 45 minutes.

Variation: Try making it with any other vegetable of your choice.

Ridge Gourd and Tomato Bake

Ingredients (Serves 4)

- 2 ridge gourds
- 2 tindas
- 3 tomatoes
- Pinch of garam masala powder
- 1/2 cup grated paneer
- A few mint leaves
- Salt and pepper to taste

Preparation

Peel and slice ridge gourds and tindas in rounds. Cut tomatoes in rings. Take a round baking dish and arrange the vegetables in layers. Sprinkle each layer with a little garam masala powder, salt, freshly ground pepper and grated paneer. Sprinkle mint leaves on top. Cover with foil and bake in an oven preheated to 190°C/ 380° F for 20-25 minutes Remove foil for the last 5 minutes of baking.

Variation: Use any other vegetable like knol khol, zuchhini, snake gourd etc. This dish can be steamed also, instead of baking.

Bitter Gourd Dry Fry

Ingredients (Serves 4)

- 1 large bitter gourd
- 1 large onion
- 1 tbsp refined oil
- Salt and pepper to taste
- 1 tsp roasted and powdered cumin seeds

Preparation

Slice both the bitter gourd and onions into thin rings. Discard tough seeds, if any. Heat the oil in a non-stick karahi and add the onion. Stir fry. When it starts to pick up brown spots, add the bitter gourd and keep stirring over high heat. Bitter gourd does not take long to cook. Add salt and pepper when done. Let the moisture evaporate. This is a dry dish. Garnish with roasted and powdered cumin. Goes well with chappatis.

Mixed Vegetables

Ingredients (Serves 4)

- 10 button mushrooms
- 50 gm French beans
- 1/2 cup shelled peas
- 100 gm baby corns
- 1 small carrot
- 1 cup shredded cabbage
- 2 large ripe tomatoes
- 1 tbsp refined oil
- 1 tsp finely chopped garlic
- 1/2 tsp grated ginger
- 1/2 tsp chopped green chilli
- 1/2 tsp salt
- 1/2 tsp pepper

Preparation

Halve the mushrooms. Cut beans and carrot into cubes. Slice the baby corns. Boil all the vegetables in 2 cups of water till tender yet crisp. Drain and reserve stock. Blanch the cabbage in 1 cup of water and drain. Blanch the tomatoes and blend to make a puree; strain. Heat the oil in a karahi. Add garlic, ginger and green chilli. Saute for 2 minutes. Add all the vegetables and 1 cup of the reserved stock. Cook for 5 minutes, then add the puree. Season with salt and pepper. Cook for another 5 minutes. Serve hot with steamed rice or chappati.

Bhuna Bhindi (Fried Okra)

Ingredients (Serves 4)

- 300 gm okra
- 50 gm curd
- 1/2 tsp coriander powder
- 1/2 tsp cumin powder
- 1/2 tsp chilli powder
- 1/2 tsp chaat masala
- 1 tsp lime juice
- 1 tbsp refined oil
- 1 medium onion, finely chopped
- 1/2 tsp grated ginger
- 1/2 tsp green chilli, chopped,
- Pinch of turmeric powder
- 1/2 tsp salt

Preparation

Take tender okras. Wash and dry well. Cut a slice off the tops and slit, but do not slit through. Mix together the coriander, cumin, chilli and chaat masala powders, lime juice and 1/2 tsp oil. Stuff the okras with this. Heat the oil in a non-stick skillet and add the onion. Saute 2 minutes. Add ginger, green chilli and turmeric. Cook for a couple of minutes. Beat the curd and add along with the salt. Mix well. Add the okras and remaining spices, if any. Cook over a medium heat for 5-10 minutes, stirring from time to time till done. There should be no gravy. Dry any excess moisture. Serve hot with rotis.

Methi Dhoka In Gravy

Ingredients (Serves 6)

- 1 cup Bengal gram dal
- 1/2 cup arhar dal
- 1 tbsp grated coconut
- 1 green chilli
- 1/2 tsp salt
- 4 tbsp fresh coriander leaves, chopped
- $1\frac{1}{2}$ cup finely chopped fenugreek leaves
- 1/2 cup sprouted moong
- 1/2 tsp sodium bicarbonate

For Gravy

- 3 tbsp Bengal gram dal
- 2 tbsp grated coconut
- 1 cm piece of ginger
- 1/2 tsp salt
- A handful of fresh coriander
- 1 tomato
- 1/2 tsp turmeric
- Pinch of asafoetida
- 1/2 tsp cumin seeds
- 1 tbsp refined oil
- 1/2 tsp mustard seeds
- 1 cup curd

Preparation

Soak the dals for 4-5 hours. Grind coarsely along with coconut, green chilli, salt and half the fresh coriander, using very little water. Add the chopped fenugreek leaves, the remaining coriander leaves and sprouted moong to the ground dal and 1/4 tsp soda; mix thoroughly. The mixture should be of pouring consistency. If necessary, add a little water. Grease a plate and pour in the batter. Steam in a pressure cooker or dhokla steamer for 20 minutes. Cool and cut into squares.

Gravy: Soak the gram dal for 2 hrs. Grind the gram dal, grated coconut, ginger, salt, coriander leaves, tomato, asafoetida and cumin into a fine paste. Heat the oil in a karahi and add mustard seeds. When it stops spluttering, add the dal paste alongwith 2 cups of water. When it comes to a boil, add the beaten curd; if necessary add more water. Let cook over a slow flame for 10 minutes. Add the steamed dhokas and cook for 2 minutes. There should be a thick gravy. Garnish with coriander leaves and serve hot.

Ayurveda recommends bitter food. Bitter taste provides an excellent balance for heavy foods - salty, sweet and sour in taste. Bitter greens like methi can lighten and enliven a meal, as well as provide generous amounts of vitamin A, iron, calcium, magnesium and other nutrients.

Pulisu

Ingredients (Serves 4)

- 4 drumsticks
- 200 gm bottle gourd
- 200 gm potatoes
- 200 gm brinjals
- 200 gm okra
- 1 tbsp tamarind paste
- 1 tsp turmeric powder
- Salt to taste

For Tempering

- 1 tbsp refined oil
- 1/2 tsp fenugreek seeds
- 1/2 tsp mustard seeds
- 1/2 tsp urad dal
- 2 red chillies
- 1 sprig curry leaves

Roast and powder

- 1 tsp coriander seeds
- 1/2 tsp asafoetida
- 2 tbsp Bengal gram dal
- 2 tsp rice
- 2 red chillies

Preparation

Soak the tamarind in a cup of water. Cut the vegetables in medium pieces. Cook them in 3 cups of water adding turmeric and salt. When the vegetables are done, mash them to form a thick gravy. Now, add the tamarind paste and cook further. Lastly add the powdered masala. Heat the oil in a separate pan. Add fenugreek and mustard seeds along with the urad dal, red chillies and curry leaves. Fry till crisp. Pour over the vegetables. Boil for a couple of minutes and remove.

Variation: Tinda and bottle gourd may be added.

Drumsticks are a wonder food. Almost all parts of the drumstick tree have therapeutic value. The pods have antiseptic value and can be used most beneficially by a diabetic.

Drumstick Curry

Ingredients (Serves 6)

- 4 drumsticks
- 2 tomatoes
- 2 green chillies
- 3 onions
- 2 cups gramflour
- 1 tbsp unsaturated oil
- 1 tsp cumin seeds
- 1 tsp mustard seeds
- 1/2 tsp turmeric powder
- 1/2 cup chopped fresh coriander
- Salt to taste

Preparation

Peel and cut the drumsticks in finger length pieces. Chop the tomatoes and green chillies. Slice the onions. Sieve the gramflour and mix with 5 cups of water. There should be no lumps. Boil drumsticks till tender with a pinch of salt. Heat the oil in a karahi. Add cumin and mustard seeds; when they pop, add onion and cook till translucent. Add tomato, green chillies and turmeric. Add the besan mixture, and a little salt and stir well till blended and cooked. Add water, if needed. Put in the drumsticks and simmer for 5 minutes over a low heat. Garnish with coriander leaves.

The drumsticks and its leaves are particularly beneficial in the treatment of a lot of ailments including diabetes due to its medicinal properties and rich iron content.

Sprouted Methi Curry

Ingredients (Serves 2)

- 1/2 cup fenugreek seeds, sprouted
- 3 medium tomatoes
- 2 tsp mustard oil
- 1/2 tsp cumin seeds
- 1/2 tsp fenugreek seeds
- 1 tsp dry ginger powder
- Salt and pepper to taste

Preparation

To sprout fenugreek seeds, soak the seeds overnight. Wash well and tie in a muslin cloth. Keep covered in a warm place for 24 hours. The seeds will sprout. Wash and chop the tomatoes. Blend in mixie till pureed. Strain. Heat the oil in a pan. Season with cumin and fenugreek seeds. When they pop up, lower heat and add the ginger powder, salt and pepper - mixed with 2 tbsp water. Stir fry till the water dries up. Add the tomato puree and sprouted seeds. Cook for 2 minutes till well blended. Serve with chappatis.

Fenugreek with its pungent and pleasant taste should be a lifelong friend of the diabetic.

STUFFED TOMATO

Ingredients (Serves 4)

- 1 cup cooked rice
- 4 large tomatoes
- 1 small onion
- 1 spring onion
- 2 cloves of garlic
- 1 small carrot
- 1 tbsp refined oil
- 1/2 tsp salt
- 1/2 tsp pepper
- 1 tbsp tomato ketchup
- 1 tsp chilli sauce

Preparation

Cut a slice off the top of the tomatoes. Discard pith and seeds. Reserve the caps. Finely chop the onion, spring onion, garlic and carrot. Heat the oil in a karahi. Add garlic. Add all the vegetables except tomato. Stir fry till soft. Add the rice, salt, pepper and ketchup. Saute for 2 minutes. Mix chilli sauce and remove. Steam the tomatoes for a minute. Stuff the tomatoes with the rice mix. Put the caps back on the tomatoes and bake in a moderate oven for 5 minutes.

Variation: Use capsicum instead. The rice tastes very good by itself also.

Savoury Cheesecake

Ingredients (Serves 4)

- 1 cup shelled peas
- 4 large cauliflower florets
- 1 medium carrot
- 1 cup paneer, grated
- 3/4 tsp salt
- Freshly ground pepper to taste
- 1 tbsp fresh coriander leaves
- 1 large tomato

For White sauce

- 2 cups skimmed milk
- 2 tbsp flour

Preparation

Boil the peas, mash coarsely. Grate the cauliflower and carrot.

White sauce: Bring the milk and flour to boil. Stir well, there should be no lumps. Add the peas, cauliflower, carrot, salt and pepper. Cover and cook till thick. Mix the paneer and remove from heat. Grease a baking dish very lightly and pour in the vegetable mixture. Bake in an oven preheated to 200°C/400°F for 15-20 minutes. Garnish with coriander leaves and tomato slices.

South Indian Style Broccoli

Ingredients (Serves 4)

- 4 cups broccoli florets
- 1 red capsicum
- 1 medium onion
- 1 tbsp sesame seeds
- 1 tbsp refined oil
- 1/2 tsp mustard seeds
- 1 tsp cumin seeds
- 1 tsp urad dal
- 8-10 curry leaves

Preparation

Wash and chop the broccoli florets into small pieces. Deseed and cube the capsicum. Slice the onion. Roast the sesame seeds. Heat the oil in a skillet and temper with the mustard seeds, urad dal and curry leaves. When the urad dal turns brown, add the onion. Fry till pink. Add the vegetables and stir fry for 2 minutes. Remove and garnish with the roasted sesame seeds.

The exotic continental vegetables are easily available these days. Make use of them.

Turnip and Radish Dal

Ingredients (Serves 2-3)

- 1 tender turnip
- 1 small tender radish
- 1/2 cup gram dal
- 2 tsp refined oil
- 1 tsp mustard seeds
- Pinch of asafoetida
- 1/2 tsp curry powder
- 3/4 tsp sea salt
- 2 tsp grated ginger
- 1 green chilli, slit
- 1/4 tsp turmeric powder

Preparation

Peel and cut the turnip and radish into small dices. Cook the dal in 2 cups of water in a pressure cooker for 8 minutes. Heat the oil in a karahi. Add the mustard seeds, when they pop, add the asafoetida, turmeric, turnip and radish. Then add the rest of the ingredients, saute 2 minutes. Cover and cook oven a medium heat for 5 minutes, adding half cup of water. Check when done. Stir fry to evaporate excess moisture, if any. Add the cooked dal and boil for 5 minutes. Serve with chappatis

In Bengal, we use what is called 'matar dal' - a kind of yellow split dal. You can substitute gram dal.

Pumpkin Treat

Ingredients (Serves 4)

- 200 gm long beans
- 1/2 kg pumpkin
- 1 tbsp refined oil
- 1/2 tsp mustard seeds
- 1/2 tsp finely chopped garlic
- 3/4 tsp sea salt
- 1 tsp coriander powder
- 1 tsp cumin powder
- 1/2 tsp curry powder

Preparation

Wash and dry the beans. Chop in 2.5 cm pieces. Wash the pumpkin, peel and slice in 1 cm thick pieces. Heat the oil in a non-stick skillet. Add the mustard and fenugreek seeds. When they pop up, put in the asafoetida, garlic and beans. Cook over a medium heat for 5 minutes. Then add the sliced pumpkins, salt and the spices. Cook, stirring for a couple of minutes. Add 1/2 cup of water; cover and cook till done. In case there is any water left, evaporate over high heat. Serve with chappatis.

Dal Dhokli

Ingredients (Serves 4)

For Dhokli

- 1 cup atta
- 1 pinch salt
- 1/2 tsp turmeric powder
- 1 tsp ajwain

For Dal

- 1 cup arhar dal
- 1 tsp turmeric
- 1/2 tsp chilli powder (optional)
- 1 tsp coriander powder
- 2 tsp tamarind pulp
- 1/2 tsp jaggery
- 1 tsp finely chopped ginger
- 8-10 curry leaves
- 1 green chilli, finely chopped

For Tempering

- 2 tsp refined oil
- 1 tsp mustard seeds
- 1/2 tsp fenugreek seeds
- A pinch of asafoetida
- Coriander leaves for garnishing

Preparation

Dhokli: Knead the atta with all the ingredients like chappati dough. Roll into thin chappatis. Cut into small pieces. Reserve.

Dal: Pressure cook the dal with the turmeric and chilli powders if using, coriander powder and 4 cups of water for 10 minutes. Mash the dal while still hot, to blend well. Add the tamarind paste, ginger, curry leaves, jaggery and green chilli, and cook for 2 minutes. Add the dhoklis and boil for 5 minutes. Add the seasoning, garnish with coriander leaves and serve hot.

Tempering: Heat the oil in a small frying pan. Add the mustard seeds, fenugreek seeds and asafoetida,. When they stop crackling add to the dal.

This Gujarati dish amounts to a one-dish meal, full of carbohydrate, protein and fibre.

Dal Fry

Ingredients (Serves 6-8)

- 300 gm mixed dals
- 2 tomatoes
- 1 onion
- 1 tsp grated ginger
- 1/2 tsp turmeric powder
- 1/2 tsp chilli powder
- 1/2 tsp cumin powder
- 1 tsp salt
- 1 tsp paanch phoran
- 1 green chilli, chopped

Preparation

Dals include masoor, moong, gram dal, arhar, moth, lobia and rajma. The dals should be of the same quantity. Soak the dals for 4 hours. Pressure cook with enough water and the turmeric for 10 minutes. Open cooker. Add the onion and tomatoes, finely chopped, ginger, chilli and cumin. Boil for 5-6 minutes. Dry roast the paanch phoran in a karahi. When they change colour and emit an aroma, pour over the dal. Cook for 5 minutes. Remove from heat and keep covered till serving time.

Knol Khol Keema

Ingredients (Serves 4)

- 400 gm knol khol (ganth gobhi)
- 1 large potato
- 1 tsp turmeric
- 1/2 tsp chilli powder
- 1/2 tsp cumin powder
- 1/2 tsp coriander powder
- 1 tsp salt
- 1/2 tsp garam masala powder
- 2 bay leaves
- 1/2 tsp paanch phoran
- 2 cinnamon sticks
- 2 tsp refined oil

Preparation

Boil the potato. Peel and cut into small cubes. Discard the leaves of the knol khol. Wash, peel and cut into halves. Grate the knol khols as you grate coconut. Heat the oil in a non-stick karahi, add the bay leaves, paanch phoran and cinnamon. When they emit their aromas, add the rest of the ingredients. Stir fry, sprinkle a little water in between. The knol khol cooks quite quickly. If the potatoes disintegrate somewhat, don't worry. This is how it should be. Garnish with coriander leaves and serve hot with chappatis.

Variation: Radish, grated can be cooked the same way.

Tomato Chutney

Ingredients

- 900 gm green tomatoes
- 1 large onion
- 1 large cooking apple
- 300 ml malt vinegar
- 1 tsp pickling spices
- 60 gm raisins
- 1/2 tsp salt
- Sugar-free sweetener equivalent to 285 gm sugar

Preparation

Pickling spices mean mustard seeds, kalonji, peppercorns 1 tsp each and 1 dry red chilli. Tie in a muslin cloth. Roughly chop the tomatoes, and onion. Peel and chop the apple. Put the vegetables and apple into a saucepan with half the vinegar and the spices. Simmer gently until they start to become soft. Add the remainder of the vinegar gradually. Then add the remaining ingredients and cook until soft and pulpy. Remove the spices and while still hot pour into sterilised jars. Will keep for at least 2-3 months.

Papaya Chutney

Ingredients (Serves 4)

- 2 cups grated raw papaya
- Sugar free sweetener equivalent to 1 tbsp sugar
- 1 tsp grated 'aam-ada'.
- Pinch of salt
- Juice of one lime

Preparation

Wash the raw papaya. Peel and remove the seeds and grate. Do not wash thereafter. This should measure 2 cups, full. Pressure cook the papaya with a pinch of salt, without water for one minute, strain; but do not discard the water. Boil the papaya water with sugar free sweetener. Add the cooked papaya and 'aam-ada' and let cook. When the water almost evaporates, add the lime juice and remove. Chill and serve.

'Aam-ada' is a ginger-like root with the aroma of raw mango, known as 'manga inji' down south. Used extensively in Bengali cooking. It is cooling and uplifts even the most jaded appetite.

Main Dish–Non Vegetarian

Sausage Risotto

Ingredients (Serves 4)

- 350 gm brown rice
- 8 chicken sausages
- 1 large onion
- 100 gm button mushrooms
- 4 tomatoes
- 1 cup shelled peas
- 2 tsp refined oil
- 3 tbsp stock
- 1 tbsp tomato ketchup
- 1 tbsp Worcestershire sauce
- 1 large tomato, quartered
- Parsley sprigs

Preparation

Cook the rice and reserve. Grill the sausages and slice. Chop the onion; slice the mushroom, quarter the tomatoes and boil the peas. Heat the oil in a non-stick karahi. Add the sausages and stock and cook for 2-3 minutes. Add the onion and cook gently until transparent. Stir in the mushroom and tomatoes and continue to cook for 5 minutes. Add the peas, rice, ketchup, Worcestershire sauce, adding a little more stock, if necessary. Cook until heated through, stirring. Taste and adjust seasonings. Turn on to a serving dish. Garnish with tomato quarters and parsley sprigs.

Brown rice, easily available in the market, has more flavour than white rice and has a higher vitamin and mineral content.

Mexican Pie

Ingredients (Serves 2)

- 150 gm boneless chicken, diced
- 1 large tomato, diced
- 1/2 cup chopped onion
- 1/2 cup chopped capsicum
- 1/2 cup cooked corn kernels
- 1 clove garlic, minced
- 1/2 tsp chilli powder
- 1/4 tsp cumin powder
- Salt to taste
- 2 tsp refined oil
- 1/2 cup grated paneer

For Crust

- 1/2 cup makki ka atta
- 1/2 cup chicken stock
- Pinch of cumin powder
- Dash of chilli powder

Preparation

Heat the oil in a non-stick skillet. Add the chicken pieces. Saute over medium heat until browned on all sides, about 5 minutes. Add the rest of the ingredients, except paneer. Lower heat, cook stirring for 5 minutes. Lightly grease a baking dish. Transfer the chicken mixture and top with the paneer. In the meantime, bring the stock (make sure it has no fat in it) to a boil in a saucepan. Stir in the makki ka atta, cumin and chilli powder. Lower heat and cook while stirring continually until the mixture thickens, say about 3 minutes. Immediately pour this on top of the paneer in the baking dish. Smoothen and make sure the topping is evenly distributed. Bake in an oven preheated to 200°C/400° F for 20-25 minutes or until the topping is golden brown and the filling bubbling. Serve hot.

This dish is inspired by Mexican tamale pie. The casserole can be made ahead, covered tightly and refrigerated, ready to bake the next day. If refrigerated take out 30 minutes before baking to bring to room temperature or add an extra 10-15 minutes to the baking time.

CHICKEN GUMBO

Ingredients (Serves 4)

- 500 gm chicken
- 3 medium onions
- 2 tomatoes
- 250 gm okra
- 5 cups chicken stock
- 1/2 tsp salt
- 1/2 tsp pepper
- 1 tsp grated ginger
- 2 cloves of garlic, finely chopped
- 1 tbsp refined oil

Preparation

Cut the chicken into pieces. Finely chop the onions and tomatoes. Wash and wipe the okras, cut a thin slice off the tops. Do not wash any further. If you refrigerate the stock for a couple of hours, you'll find the fat congealed on top. Lift out and discard. Pressure cook the chicken with the stock, onion, tomato, salt, pepper, ginger and garlic for 5 minutes. When cool, take out the chicken pieces and discard the bones. Heat the oil in a degchi and fry the okras for 3-4 minutes. Put the soup to boil. Add the boneless chicken and okras. Cook till the okras are done. Serve hot.

Khow Suey

Ingredients (Serves 4)

- 1 large onion
- 1 cup small pieces of noodles
- 2 tbsp atta
- 1 egg
- 8 pieces of chicken
- 2 cups thin coconut milk
- 1/2 tsp salt
- 1 tsp lime juice
- Few cornflakes

Preparation

Slice the onion. Roast the atta to a light brown. Hard boil the egg. Pressure cook the chicken with 2 cups of water. Debone and shred the flesh. Reserve the stock. Mix the coconut milk with the atta and add to the chicken and stock. Add the noodles, salt and pepper. Boil for 5-7 minutes. The noodles should be well done. Serve in individual bowls garnished with the chopped hardboiled eggs. Sprinkle the lime juice and cornflakes on top.

It is a popular Burmese dish, adapted to suit the diabetic diet.

Bologness Sauce

Ingredients (Serves 2)

- 1 tbsp extra virgin olive oil
- 1 medium onion, finely chopped
- 100 gm minced mutton
- 1 small carrot, grated
- 3 tsp soya sauce
- 4-5 large tomatoes
- 1 cup of water
- 1 tbsp tomato puree
- 1 heaped tsp atta mixed with a little water
- Freshly ground pepper to taste
- 1/4 tsp grated nutmeg

Preparation

Blanch the tomatoes, peel and chop roughly. Heat the oil in a non-stick skillet. Add onion and stir fry gently for about 5 minutes till soft and translucent. Add the mince and fry till brown. Put in the carrot, soya sauce, tomatoes, water and tomato puree. Stir well. Bring to the boil, then lower heat. Cover and simmer for 20-25 minutes, stirring occasionally. Stir in the atta and bring back to the boil. Stir for a minute and season with pepper and nutmeg. The sauce must be thick. Serve hot with pasta. Goes well with chappatis, too.

This tasty mince and tomato sauce is invariably associated with pasta. Real Bolognese sauce is rather rich and includes liver, wine and cream. This version is simpler and more easily digested. Just the thing for a diabetic.

CHICKEN CHINESE STYLE

Ingredients (Serves 2)

- 150 gm boneless chicken
- 1 tbsp soya sauce
- 1 tsp chilli sauce
- 75 gm flat beans (sem)
- 1 tsp cornflour
- 2 tbsp water
- 350 ml water

Preparation

Cut the chicken into narrow strips and marinate in a mixture of soya sauce and chilli sauce for 30 minutes. String the beans and cut into strips lengthwise. Combine cornflour and 2 tbsp water. Reserve. Bring the water to a boil in a karahi and add the chicken pieces. Cover and cook till tender over a low heat. There should be a cup of water left. When the chicken is done. If necessary, add some more hot water. Add the flat beans and continue cooking for 2 minutes more. The beans should retain their crispness. Add the reserved cornflour and continue to cook and stir until all the ingredients are well glazed. Serve over boiled noodles.

Chicken in Lemon Sauce

Ingredients (Serves 5)

- 1 chicken, approximately 1 kg
- 1 large capsicum
- 2 tbsp kasuri methi
- 1 tsp salt
- 1 tsp pepper
- 1 tsp garlic paste
- 2 tbsp lime juice
- 1 tsp grated lime rind
- 1/2 cup of water
- 6 wedges of lime for garnishing

Preparation

Remove the skin and cut chicken curry style, that is in 15-16 pieces. Deseed and slice the capsicum in long strips. Dry roast the kasuri methi lightly and powder coarsely. Mix the salt, pepper and garlic paste and rub all over the chicken. Place in a baking dish. Combine the capsicum, lime juice, lime rind and water. Pour half of this over the chicken. Sprinkle the kasuri methi powder over it. Bake in an oven preheated to 200° C/ 400° F for 20 minutes. Brush the chicken with the remaining sauce and bake for another 20 minutes or until the chicken is done. Garnish with lemon wedges and serve.

Chick Peas and Chicken

Ingredients (Serves 2)

- 100 gm chick peas
- 300 ml water
- 300 ml apple juice
- 2 cloves of garlic, crushed
- 2 bay leaves
- 1/2 tsp cumin powder
- 200 g boneless chicken cubes
- Salt and pepper to taste
- 2 tbsp cornmeal (makki ka atta)

Preparation

Soak the chick peas overnight. Pressure cook with the water for 10 minutes. The chick peas should not to be fully cooked. Drain. Mix the chick peas with all the ingredients together except the cornmeal. Cook in a pressure cooker for 10 minutes. Mix the cornmeal with a little water. Add to the chick peas. Simmer for 5 minutes till the gravy thickens.

Variation: If you do not want to use the apple juice, use water instead.

Dried beans and legumes—eg., chick peas have dietary fibres and roughage which helps to lower blood sugar levels. So do try to incorporate them in your diet as often as you can.

Chappati Float

Ingredients (Serves 4)

For Floats

- 1 cup atta,
- A pinch of salt
- 4-5 spring onions, finely chopped
- 1/3 cup fresh coriander leaves

For Topping

- 1 cup thick curd
- 1 small cucumber, deseeded and grated
- 1 tsp garlic paste
- A pinch of salt

For Sauce

- 250 gm chicken mince
- 1 cup thick tomato puree
- 1 cup water
- 1/4 tsp each of salt and pepper

Preparation

Floats: Mix the atta and salt and knead to a dough, like chappati. Divide into balls. Roll into thin puri like circles. Cut into neat squares. Mix onion and fresh coriander. Take one square, fill with the onion mixture. Cover with another square and pinch edges to seal. Prepare all others the same way. Boil enough water in a large pan. Add the floats. Remove with a slotted spoon when done. Put in a serving plate.

Mince Sauce: Put all the ingredients to boil together. Cook till the mince is done and thick. Pour the mince sauce over the floats. Cover with the curd topping, garnish with coriander.

Topping: Whip the curd and mix the cucumber, garlic paste and salt.

Rajasthani Meat

Ingredients (Serves 4)

- 500 gm lean, boneless mutton
- 1/2 cup curd
- 1 tsp salt
- 2 tsp oil

Grind together

- 1 large onion
- 6 cloves of garlic
- 2 green chillies
- 1 tsp white peppercorns
- 1 tsp cumin seeds
- 3 tbsp poppy seeds
- 2 tbsp pumpkin seeds (magaj)

Preparation

Trim all visible fat and cut mutton into bite-sized cubes. Heat the oil in a non-stick saucepan. Add the ground paste and stir fry for 5 minutes on low heat. Add the mutton, salt and 1 cup of water. Cover and cook over a low heat till done and the gravy thick.

It is an exotic party dish, cooked the diabetic way.

MUTTON BHOPLA

Ingredients (Serves 3)

- 6 pieces of mutton, 100 gms each
- 6 large pieces of ash gourd
- 1 onion
- 1 clove garlic
- 1 green chilli
- 1 small piece of ginger
- 1 pinch turmeric powder
- 1 pinch of powdered garam masala
- 1/4 cup curd
- 1 bay leaf
- 1 tbsp refined oil
- Salt to taste

Preparation

Beat the curd and marinate the meat in it for one hour. Grind together the onion, ginger, garlic, turmeric and green chilli. You may omit the chilli, if you wish. Heat the oil in a non-stick skillet and add the ground paste. When you get a fried aroma, add the garam masala powder, meat, bay leaf and cook, stirring. Once the oil separates, add hot water. Cover and cook. In the meantime, peel and cook the pumpkin till soft. Prepare a puree by straining. Add the cooked mutton and let cook for a further 5 minutes. There should be a thick gravy. Garnish with coriander and serve.

The ash gourd or 'petha' as it is known in Hindi is diuretic, cooling and relaxes the body.

Chicken–Do–Piaza

Ingredients (Serves 6)

- 1 kg chicken
- 1 tsp turmeric powder
- 1 tsp cumin powder
- 1/2 tsp ginger paste
- 1/2 tsp garlic paste
- 1 tsp soya sauce
- 1 tsp Worcestershire sauce
- 2 tbsp refined oil
- 3 capsicums
- 2 onions
- 1 tsp cumin seeds
- Tomato slices for garnishing

Preparation

Cut the chicken in pieces. Mix all the spices, soya sauce, Worcestershire sauce and 1 tbsp oil, marinate the chicken in it for half an hour. Cut the capsicum and onion into square pieces. Heat 1 tablespoon oil in a non stick karahi. Add the cumin seeds. Add the chicken and fry well for 5 minutes. Add onion and capsicum. Stir fry 2 minutes. Add water, cover and cook till done. Taste and add salt, if needed. The sauces are quite salty. There should be a little gravy. Serve with chappati, garnished with tomato slices.

Haleem

Ingredients (Serves 6)

- 250 gm boneless mutton
- 1/4 cup gram dal
- 1/4 cup moong dal
- 1/4 cup masur dal
- 1/4 cup wheat
- 1/2 tsp turmeric powder
- 1 tsp salt
- 1 tbsp ginger paste
- 1 tsp garlic paste
- 1/2 tsp coriander powder
- 2 tbsp refined oil
- 2 large onions, sliced
- 1 tomato, chopped
- 1/3 cup curd
- Pinch of garam masala powder
- Coriander leaves for garnishing

Preparation

The mutton should be lean. Discard fat, if any. Pressure cook the dals and wheat (dalia may be used instead) with turmeric and salt for 10 minutes. Marinate the mutton in ginger - garlic paste and coriander and cumin powders for half an hour. Pressure cook the mutton with 3 cups of water for 15 minutes. Heat the oil in a degchi. Add the onion and fry till light brown. Add chopped tomato and whipped curd. Fry for 5 minutes till the tomatoes soften and stir well. Add the cooked dal, mutton and garam masala powder. Boil for 10 minutes on low heat till everything is well mixed. Garnish with chopped coriander leaves.

STEAMED CHUTNEY FISH

Ingredients (Serves 4)

- 4 thick bhetki fillets
- 1 pinch of salt
- Juice of 1 lime
- 4 large pieces of banana leaves

Grind to a paste

- 2 tsp grated coconut
- 1/3 cup chopped coriander leaves
- 6-8 mint leaves
- Pinch of sugar
- 1 tsp lime juice
- 2 green chillies
- 1 tsp grated ginger

Preparation

Slit the fillets from one side, but do not slit through. It should form a pocket. Marinate in salt and lime juice for 1 hour. Stuff the chutney inside the fish and coat the outsides as well. Keep aside for at least an hour. Take 4 large pieces of banana leaves. Keep one fish on each leaf. Wrap well and tie with string. Steam for 25-30 minutes or till done. Can be baked also. In that case grease the outside of the leaves a little. The packets can be roasted on a tava till the leaves get charred. If you can't get banana leaves, use aluminum foils instead. But the particular delicious flavour imparted by the banana leaves gets lost.

Light, but filling; a diabetic's delight.

Machher Jhal
(Bengali Fish Curry I)

Ingredients (Serves 4)

- 500 gm fish, pomfret, mackarel, bhetki or rohu
- $1\frac{1}{2}$ tbsp mustard oil
- 1 tsp fenugreek seeds
- 1/2 tsp turmeric powder
- 1/2 tsp garlic paste
- 200 gm tomatoes, finely chopped
- 1 tsp salt
- 1/2 cup of water
- 4 green chillies, slit
- 1/2 tsp chilli powder
- 1 cup finely chopped fresh coriander

Preparation

Wash the fish well. Heat 1 tbsp oil in a karahi. Add the fenugreek seeds. When they stop spluttering and get fragrant add the turmeric, chilli, garlic paste, tomatoes and salt. Cook over a medium heat till the tomatoes are soft and the raw smell of garlic disappears. Add the water and green chillies. When it comes to a boil add the fish and cook till done. Add the coriander leaves and 1/2 tbsp of raw mustard oil. Remove and serve with boiled rice.

Fish in Curd

Ingredients (Serves 4)

- 8 pieces of rohu, katla or bhetki
- 1/2 cup of fresh curd
- 1/2 tsp turmeric powder
- $1^1/_2$ tsp ground ginger
- 2 green chillies, slit
- 1 large onion, grated
- 1/2 tsp salt
- 1 tbsp white mustard seeds
- 1 bay leaf
- 10 peppercorns
- 1/2 tsp garam masala powder

Preparation

Wash the fish well. Whip the curd and add to it the turmeric, grated ginger, green chillies, onion, salt and mustard paste. Marinate the fish in it for 1 hour. Dry roast the bay leaves and peppercorns in a karahi. When they become fragrant, add the fish along with the marinade and 1/2 cup of water. Cook over a high heat till it comes to a boil. Lower heat and cover. Simmer till the fish is done and the gravy thickens a bit. Sprinkle with garam masala and remove.

It is a delicacy from Bengal, adapted to suit a diabetic diet and is totally oil free.

Machher Jhol
(Bengali Fish Curry II)

Ingredients (Serves 4)

- 1/2 kg fish
- 1 tsp turmeric powder
- 1 small potato
- 4 parwals
- 1 small brinjal
- 4 flat beans (sem)
- 1 heaped tsp aniseed
- 1 cm piece of ginger
- 1 tbsp mustard oil
- 1/2 tsp paanch phoran
- 3/4 tsp salt
- 2 green chillies, slit

Preparation

Wash fish, smear with half the turmeric. Keep aside. Peel and cut the potato into fingers. Peel at intervals and cut the parwals into two. Cut the brinjal in small pieces. Top, tail and string the flat beans, keeping them whole. Grind the aniseed and ginger. Heat the oil in a karahi, temper with the paanch phoran. When they emit an aroma, add the vegetables and stir fry for 2 minutes. Add the turmeric, ground spices and stir for 2 minutes more. Add enough water to cook the vegetables, add salt. Cover. When the vegetables are 3/4 done, add the fish and green chillis. The gravy is soupy so add water accordingly. Cook till the fish is done. *Variation:* Use any other vegetable like ridge gourd, raw papaya, drumstick, etc.

This very light stew-like fish curry from Bengal uses aniseed paste. Aniseed, or saunf is cooling, appetising and has a digestive enzyme. This fish curry should be a staple for the diabetic during summer.

Fish with Mustard Paste

Ingredients (Serves 2)

- 100 gm rohu
- Juice of 1 lime
- 1/2 tsp salt
- 3 tsp refined oil or mustard oil
- 2 onions
- 1 cm piece of ginger
- 2 cloves of garlic
- 2 green chillies
- 1 tbsp mustard seeds
- 1/2 tsp turmeric powder
- A handful of coriander leaves

Preparation

Cut the fish in 4 pieces. Wash well. Marinate in lime juice and salt for 15 minutes. Lightly fry in very little oil. A non-stick pan helps. (This oil is extra). Finely chop onion, ginger, garlic and green chillies. Grind the mustard seeds to a fine paste. Heat 2 tsp oil in a karahi, add onion and stir fry for 2 minutes. Add ginger paste and saute for another couple of minutes. Add 1 cup of water, turmeric and mustard paste. When it comes to a boil, add the fish, a little salt and coriander leaves. Boil for 2 minutes more. Finally sprinkle the remaining 1 tsp raw mustard oil and remove. Serve hot.

Fish Loaf

Ingredients (Serves 4)

- 500 gm fish
- 2-3 large slices of brown bread
- 2 cups cooked noodles
- 2 green chillies
- 1 cm piece of ginger
- 1/4 tsp grated nutmeg
- 1/2 tsp roasted and powdered cumin
- 2 cubes cheese, grated (optional)
- 2 eggs
- 1 cup milk
- 1/3 cup chopped fresh coriander leaves
- 1/2 tsp salt
- 1 large tomato, finely chopped
- 1 onion, grated

Preparation

Any large fish like rohu, bhetki, pomfret or surmai will do. Steam fish; remove bones and flake. Process the bread slices to make fresh bread crumbs. Grind ginger and green chillies together. Mix together all the ingredients and put in a lightly greased baking dish. Bake in an oven preheated to 180°C/350°F for one hour or till a knife inserted in the middle comes out clean.

Stuffed Fish

Ingredients (Serves 4)

- 1 whole bhetki fish, approx 500-600 gm
- 1 tbsp lime juice
- 1/2 tsp salt

For stuffing

- 250 gm chicken mince
- 2 large onions, finely chopped
- 1 tbsp ginger-garlic paste
- 1/2 tsp pepper
- 2 tbsp Worcestershire sauce

For Topping

- $1^1/_2$ cups curd
- 1/2 tsp salt
- Pinch of chilli powder
- 1 tbsp refined oil
- $1^1/_2$ tsp cumin seeds

Preparation

Keep the fish whole. Debone. Clean the insides. Wash well. Ask your fish seller to do it for you. Smear the fish inside out with the lime juice and salt. Marinate for 20 minutes.

Stuffing: Mix all the ingredients together except oil and marinate for 20 minutes. Heat the oil and add the mince. Stir fry over high heat for 2 minutes. Cover and let cook in its own steam. If necessary, add a tbsp or two of water. Uncover when the mince is done. Dry away excess moisture, if any. Keep aside. Beat the curd and mix salt and chilli powder. Smear the fish with a little of the curd mixture. Stuff the mince inside the fish. Place on a baking dish. Pour over the rest of the curd mixture. Heat the oil and temper with the cumin seeds. When the seeds stop popping, sprinkle over the fish. Bake in an oven preheated to 180°C/350°F for about 20 -25 minutes.

Poached Mackarel

Ingredients (Serves 4)

- 6 pieces of mackarel or pomfret
- 1 cup of water
- 3 tbsp white vinegar
- 1 bay leaf
- 2 onions, cut into rings
- 10 peppercorns
- 5 cloves
- 2 cloves of garlic
- 1/2 tsp salt
- 1 tbsp parsley or fresh coriander
- 1 tsp cornflour

Preparation

Wash the fish well. Put in the water, vinegar and bay leaf in a non-stick skillet. Lay the fish pieces side by side. Cover with the onion rings, pepper, cloves, garlic and salt. Cover and cook over a moderate heat till the fish is done. Take out the fish carefully onto a serving plate and keep warm. Mix the cornflour with 2 tbsp of the stock; add to the pan. Boil till the gravy is a little thick. Pour over the fish. Discard the bay leaves. Garnish with parsley or coriander leaves. Serve hot with bread or chappati.

Shepherd's Pie

Ingredients (Serves 2)

For Base

- 2 medium potatoes
- 2 tbsp milk,
- Pinch of salt
- 1/2 tsp pepper

For Filling

- 4 pieces of fish
- 1 cup milk
- 1/2 cup of water
- 1$^1/_2$ tbsp gramflour or atta

For Topping

- 1 tbsp fresh coriander leaves
- 1 tbsp dry bread crumbs
- 1/2 tsp chilli powder
- 1/2 tsp pepper

Preparation

Base: Boil, peel and mash the potatoes. Add milk, salt and pepper. Mash again till well mixed.

Filling: Cook the fish in milk and water combined. Debone and flake fish. Add the gramflour or atta to the fish stock. Add the fish to it with a pinch of salt.

Finale: Take a baking dish. Line with the mashed potatoes. Place the filling in it. Combine the topping ingredients and sprinkle over the fish. Bake in a an oven preheated to 180°C/350°F for 15 minutes.

Variation: Vegetarians may use cooked soya granules or paneer.

Bottle Gourd and Fish Stew

Ingredients (Serves 4)

- 300 gm bottle gourd
- 4 pieces of fish
- 1 tbsp refined oil or mustard oil
- 1/2 tsp fenugreek seeds
- 1 pinch of turmeric powder
- 1 tsp coriander-cumin powder
- Salt to taste
- A handful of chopped coriander leaves
- 2 green chillies (optional)

Preparation

Peel and cut the gourd into 8 pieces. Any fish like rohu, katla, tangra, pabda, pomfret or surmai will do. Heat the oil in a karahi. Temper with fenugreek seeds. When these emit an aroma add the gourd and stir fry for 2 minutes. Add the turmeric, coriander - cumin powder and salt. Stir for one minute and add $1^1/_2$ cups of water. Cover and cook over a moderate heat till the gourd is done. A pressure cooker may be used also. Uncover and add the fish when the gourd is done. Cook over high heat till the fish is done. Sprinkle the coriander leaves. Add the green chillies, if using, and keep covered till serving time.

Variation: Raw papaya can be used the same way.

Bottle gourd or lauki is cooling and particularly good during summer. This stew is good to eat and easy to digest. The whole family will love it.

COUNTRY-STYLE FISH CHOWDER

Ingredients (Serves 4)

- 1/2 kg fish, cut into 8 pieces
- 8 French beans
- 4 cauliflower florets
- 1 cup shelled peas
- 1 tiny turnip
- 6 small onions
- 1 tbsp refined oil
- 4 cloves garlic, finely chopped
- 1/4 cup chopped celery
- 4 tbsp atta
- 2 bay leaves
- Salt and pepper to taste
- 6-8 sprigs parsley

Preparation

Wash fish well. Any fish like rohu, pomfret, surmai or bhetki will do. Wash and cut the vegetables into bite sized pieces. Do not wash any further. Keep the onions whole. Heat the oil in a non-stick saucepan. Add garlic; saute till fragrant. Add celery, saute for a minute. Add the atta and fry well, stirring. Add all the vegetables one by one, stir-frying after each addition. Add 6 cups of water, bay leaves, salt and freshly ground pepper. Cover and cook till the vegetables are done. Uncover and add the fish and parsley. Cook till the fish is done. There should be a semi-thick liquid. Remove bay leaves before serving.

Variation : Use chicken in place of fish.

This comforting chowder will offset the effects of a chilly day. Serve it with a crusty bread and a fresh fruit for dessert. Dinner couldn't be easier.

Macaroni Bake

Ingredients (Serves 4)

- 150 gm elbow macaroni
- 250 gm fish
- 100 gm mushrooms, sliced
- 200 gm sweet corn kernels
- 4 tbsp chopped capsicum
- 6 tbsp brown breadcrumbs
- 2 tbsp grated cheese

For Sauce

- 1 tbsp refined oil
- $4^1/_2$ tbsp atta
- 450 ml milk
- Salt and pepper to taste
- 1 tsp mustard powder
- 50 gm hung curd
- 50 gm paneer, grated

Preparation

Cook macaroni till 'al dente'—which means it should have a bite left in it after being cooked. Cook the fish till done. Remove bones and flake fish.

Sauce: heat the oil in a non-stick skillet, Remove from heat and stir in the atta until smooth. Gradually add the milk, then return to the heat and simmer for 2-3 minutes, stirring until thickened. Stir salt, pepper, mustard, hung curd and paneer and simmer for a further couple of minutes. Mix together the macaroni, mushroom, corn, capsicum and fish and toss in the sauce. Pour the mixture into an ovenproof dish. Mix the breadcrumbs and cheese and sprinkle over the top. Bake for 15-20 minutes on medium temperature. Serve as snack, supper dish or with vegetables as a main curse.

Pasta can be treted and used as a main course or snack meal or used in place of potatoes to accompany meat or fish dishes. Pasta is also delicious in soups or cooked and added to salads. Do use wholemeal pasta, if you get it.

SNACKS

TANDOORI CHICKEN

Ingredients (Serves 4)

- 8 chicken legs
- Juice of 1 lime
- 250 gm curd
- 1 tsp coriander powder
- 1 tsp cumin powder
- 1 tbsp ginger paste
- 1 tsp salt
- Freshly ground pepper to taste
- 1 tbsp raw papaya paste
- 2 tsp refined oil

Preparation

Slit the chicken legs at a few places and pat dry. Hang the curd for a couple of hours so that the whey drains. Mix the remaining ingredients except oil and marinate the chicken legs in it for at least 4 hours, preferably overnight. Bake in a gas tandoor or grill, turning often. Baste with the oil and marinade from time to time. It will take about 20-25 minutes. You'll have to do it in 2 batches. An oven can be used also, but it misses out on the smoky flavour that a tandoor imparts.

Calcutta Burgers

Ingredients (Serves 2)

- 1 green chilli
- 1 clove of garlic
- 250 gm minced chicken
- 2 tbsp finely chopped capsicum
- 1 tbsp thick tomato puree
- 3 tsp gramflour
- A pinch each of powdered coriander, cumin, chilli, dry ginger, nutmeg, cloves and cinnamon
- Salt and pepper to taste
- 2 tbsp apple juice

Preparation

Mince the green chilli and garlic together. Mix all the ingredients together except the apple juice and half and gramflour. Add enough juice to give the mixture a firm consistency. Shape into burgers and dust with the remaining gram flour. Cook under a preheated grill for 15-20 minutes, turning occasionally until browned and done. You may brush with a little oil once.

Shape the burgers thinner than regular ones, so they cook better.

Liver Spread

Ingredients (Serves 2)

- 200 gm mutton or chicken liver
- 2 large onions
- 1/4 cup vinegar
- 1/4 tsp salt
- 1 tbsp freshly ground pepper
- 1/2 tsp refined oil

Preparation

Wash the liver and pat dry. Mince coarsely with a knife. do not wash after this. Finely chop the onions. Marinate the liver in vinegar and salt for 2 hours. Heat the oil in a karahi, non-stick preferred. Add the onions and saute till pink. Add the liver mixture and quickly saute on high heat. Add pepper, mix and remove. Liver cooks quickly. Do not overcook; it becomes tough.

This makes yummy sandwich spread. Equally good with chappatis.

Double Decker Sandwich

Ingredients (Makes 4 Sandwiches)

- 1 cup thick spinach paste
- 1/4 tsp garlic paste
- Salt and pepper to taste
- 200 gm boneless chicken
- 4 hardboiled eggs
- 1/2 cup hung curd
- 12 slices brown bread

Preparation

To make the spinach paste - cook the spinach, leaves only, till wilted. Squeeze to get rid of all water. Blend to a puree. Cook over a medium fire till excess water dries up. Mix with the garlic paste and a little salt and pepper. Cook the boneless chicken till done. Divide into flakes. Mash the hardboiled eggs and mix with salt, pepper and hung curd. Trim the sides of the breads. Take one slice. Spread the spinach paste, top with a little cooked chicken. Cover with a slice of bread. Top this with egg and curd mixture. Cover with a third slice of bread. Serve wrapped in paper napkins held in place with a tooth pick.

Variation: You may add a little grated cheese or paneer with the spinach.

PITTA SANDWICH

Ingredients (Makes 16 Sandwiches)

For Dough

- 2 cups atta
- 1 tbsp fresh yeast
- 1 tsp salt
- Pinch of sugar
- 1 tsp refined oil

For Chick pea Spread

- 200 gm chick peas
- 3 cloves of garlic, crushed
- 1 tbsp lime juice
- Salt to taste

For Salad

- 1/2 cup finely shredded cabbage
- 1 spring onion, finely chopped
- 4 small tomatoes, chopped
- Salt and pepper to taste

For Pitta:

- Soak the yeast in 1/2 cup of warm water and sugar for 5 minutes

Preparation

Sift the atta on a tray and make a bay in the centre. Add the yeast mixture, salt and oil. Add enough warm water to make a soft but pliable dough. Keep covered in a warm draught free place till doubled in bulk. Punch the dough down and knead very well for 10 minutes. Divide into 8 portions. Roll out each into oblongs. Do not roll very thinly. Keep covered for 10 minutes. Preheat oven to 190°C/235°F. Bake the breads on a tray till puffed up. Alternatively, heat a tawa, put the bread on it. Turn once and allow to puff up on the gas. Slit into 2 from the middle. Let cool.

Spread: Soak the chickpeas in water for 5-6 hours. Pressure cook till done. Drain and puree in a blender. Add lime juice, salt and garlic.

To assemble: Take a pitta bread. It will have a pocket. Spread the chickpea paste inside. Stuff the salad and serve.

Variation: Use any other vegetables or a salad of your own choice.

Pitta is Greek bread. Its very easy to make your own pitta at home. I have used atta for additional nutrition.

Steamed Omelette

Ingredients (Serves 4)

- 4 eggs
- 2 tbsp cooked and flaked chicken
- 2 tbsp boiled peas
- 2 tbsp grated onion
- 1/4 tsp grated ginger
- Pinch of salt
- Freshly crushed pepper to taste

Preparation

Separate the egg yolks and whites. Beat the yolks lightly and mix the rest of the ingredients except the egg whites. Whip the egg whites till stiff. Fold into the egg yolk mixture. Lightly grease a container with a tight fitting lid. Pour in the egg mixture and steam in a pressure cooker for 5-7 minutes. Cut into pieces and serve. This can be made into a curry also.

Variation: Use fish in place of chicken or other vegetables. Rice cooker or dhokla steamer can be used for steaming.

Spiced 2 Grain Pancake

Ingredients (Makes 14 Pancakes)

- 1 cup rolled oats
- 1/4 cup toasted wheat germs
- 1 cup milk
- 1 egg
- 3/4 cup flour
- 1 tsp baking powder
- 1 1/4 tsp dry ginger powder
- 1 1/4 tsp cinnamon powder
- 1/2 tsp ground cloves
- 1 tsp salt
- Refined oil for brushing griddle

Preparation

In a blender blend all the ingredients except the oil until just combined. Heat a non-stick tawa over moderate heat until hot enough to make a drop of water scatter over surface and brush with oil. Working in batches, drop scant 1/4 cup batter into tawa. Rotate tawa to form pancakes about 10 cm in diametre and cook until bubbles appear on surface and undersides are brown, about 2 minutes. Flip pancakes with a spatula and cook until undersides are golden brown and pancakes are cooked through, about 2 minutes.

Variation: Serve with any curry of your choice. These can be stuffed with a filling of your choice and baked, too.

Tomato Frittata

Ingredients (Serves 4)

- 1 spring onion
- 2 medium tomatoes
- 1/2 cup grated cheese
- 2 eggs
- 4 basil leaves, chopped
- Salt
- Freshly ground pepper to taste
- 2 tsp refined oil

Preparation

Finely chop the spring onion, including part of the green top. Thinly slice the tomatoes. Heat the oil in a non-stick frying pan and saute the spring onion for 1 minute, until wilted. Beat the eggs lightly and add to the pan; turn the heat to medium low arrange the tomato slices in overlapping layer on top of the eggs. Cover with grated cheese. Sprinkle with basil, salt and pepper. Cook until the batter is set and the top still wet. Place the pan under the grill until the top is puffed, sizzling and set, 1-2 minutes. Remove and using a spatula slide the frittata onto a serving dish. Cut into 4 wedges. Served with a fruit salad this makes a light but satisfying meal.

Variation: Use coriander leaves if you can't get hold of basil leaves.

The beauty of this baked omelette is that it is equally delicious, hot or cold.

MUESLI

Ingredients (Serves 4)

- 60 gm dried apricots
- 60 gm raisins
- 1/2 cup rolled oats
- 1/2 cup cornflakes
- 1/2 cup puffed rice
- 1/2 cup kheel
- 60 gm cashewnuts
- 1/4 tsp mixed spice

Preparation

Chop the apricots and cashewnuts. Mix all the ingredients together and store in an airtight container. Serve with milk or curd. You may add fresh fruits and any other nuts of your choice.

Muesli is the best way to start your day with. This is an Indian version of the Swiss muesli.

GRILLED VEGETABLES WITH PANEER

Ingredients (Serves 4)

- 200 gm paneer
- 100 gm mushrooms
- 50 gm baby corn
- 1 cup shredded cabbage

Marinade

- 100 ml tomato puree
- 1 tbsp refined oil
- Pinch of salt
- Pinch of sugar
- 1 tsp white pepper powder

Preparation

Cut paneer into cubes. Boil mushrooms and baby corn until crisp tender. Drain and reserve. Mix all the marinating ingredients together and marinate the paneer and vegetables in it for at least 2 hours or more, if time permits. Pour the vegetables, paneer along with the marinade in a baking dish and grill in a preheated oven 190°C/380°F for half an hour. Remove and serve hot.

Curd Cheese Balls

Ingredients (Makes 36 Balls)

- 3 cups curd
- 1 tbsp poppy seeds
- 1 tbsp sesame seeds
- 1 tsp cumin seeds
- 1/2 tbsp coriander seeds
- 1 tsp chaat masala
- A pinch of salt
- 1 tbsp freshly ground pepper
- 3-4 tbsp finely chopped toasted nuts
- 1/3 cup finely chopped fresh coriander leaves

Preparation

To prepare curd cheese, tie the homemade curd (made from skimmed milk) in a muslin cloth and hang for 6-8 hours till all the whey drips off. You may lightly squeeze the bundle a few times to quicken the process. Refrigerate till needed. You can do this 2 days in advance. Dry roast the poppy seeds and sesame seeds separately. Roast the coriander and cumin seeds until fragrant. Crush to a coarse powder. Place the coriander and cumin powder, chaat masala, salt and pepper in a bowl. Add the curd cheese; mix well. Place the poppy seeds, sesame seeds, roasted nuts and fresh coriander leaves on 4 different plates. Divide curd cheese into 4 portions. Using a measuring spoon, scoop up about 1/2 tbsp of curd cheese and drop 9 measured portions on each of the coatings (for a total of 36 balls). Carefully roll the balls in the coating until round and well-coated. Refrigerate until needed.

Have this nutritious snack when hunger pang strikes in between meals. They make a very good party snack, too.

VERMICELLI IDLI

Ingredients (Makes 6 Idlis)

- 200 g vermicelli
- 40 g semolina
- 1 1/2 cups curd
- 1/2 cup shelled peas
- 6 French beans, finely chopped
- 3 tbsp chopped fresh coriander leaves
- 2 tbsp chopped curry leaves
- 2.5 cm piece of ginger, grated
- Pinch of soda biocarbonate
- Salt to taste
- 1 tbsp refined oil
- 1 tbsp Bengal gram dal
- 1 tsp urad dal

Preparation

Dry roast the vermicelli and semolina separately till they emit an aroma. Heat the oil in a karahi and Add the urad dal and gram dal. Fry till a light golden brown. Now, add grated ginger and curry leaves. Saute till crisp and add the peas and beans. Stir fry for a couple of minutes. Mix together the vermicelli, semolina, curd, soda, vegetable mixture, salt, fresh coriander and sufficient water to make a batter of idli consistency. Keep aside for 30 minutes. Grease idli moulds with very little oil and pour in the batter. Steam for 5 minutes. Serve with sambhar and coconut chutney.

Spinach Idli

Ingredients (Makes 10 Idlis)

- 1 cup curd
- 250 gm semolina
- 1 bunch spinach
- 1/2 tsp sodium bicarbonate
- A pinch of salt
- 1 tsp ginger-green chilli paste
- 2 tsp refined oil
- 1/4 cup paneer, grated

Preparation

Beat the curd and soak semolina in it for an hour. Wash the spinach leaves thoroughly, discarding the stems. Drain well and chop finely. Add the soda and salt. Mix well. Mix the spinach, semolina and ginger-green chilli paste. Add oil. Grease idli moulds and pour in the batter. Steam for 10 minutes. Serve the idlis on grated paneer. The paneer may be seasoned with a little chaat masala.

Spinach cooks quickly and is a concentrated source of oxalic acid. It also cools and nourishes the body.

Colocasia Leaf Patod

Ingredients (Serves 6)

- 10 colocasia leaves
- 1 $^{1}/_{2}$ cup gramflour (besan)
- 1/4 tsp salt
- 1/2 tsp turmeric powder
- 1 tsp coriander powder
- 1 tsp cumin powder
- 2 tsp sesame seeds
- 1/2 tsp bicarbonate of soda
- Pinch of asafoetida
- 1 tsp ginger-green chilli paste
- 1 tsp garam masala powder
- Pinch of sugar
- 1 tbsp tamarind juice
- 1 tbsp refined oil
- 1 tsp mustard seeds
- 2 tbsp coriander leaves
- 2 tbsp grated coconut

Preparation

Remove the thick stems of the colocasia leaves; wash and set aside. Sieve the gramflour with soda and mix with salt, turmeric, coriander and cumin powders, sesame seeds, asafoetida, ginger green chilli paste, sugar and 1 tsp oil. Add the tamarind juice and enough water to gram flour mixture to form a paste. Spread evenly on the back of each leaf. Fold over the two sides and then roll, making sure that the batter does not spill. Place the rolls on a sieve and steam. A dhokla steamer may be used as well. Steam for 45 minutes. Cut the steamed roll into thick pieces.Heat the oil in a non - stick skillet and temper with the mustard seeds. When they crackle lay the rolls side by side and leave on a low heat. After 5-7 minutes flip so the other sides are fried, too. Remove after 5 minutes, garnish with coconut and coriander leaves. Serve hot or cold.

Variation: Cabbage leaves may be used as well.

Stuffed Khandvi

Ingredients (Serves 4)

For Khandvi

- 1 cup besan
- 1 cup butter milk
- 1 tsp ginger green chilli paste
- 1/4 tsp turmeric powder
- 1/2 tsp salt

For Stuffing

- 3/4 cup shelled green peas
- 1/2 tsp ginger-green chilli paste
- Pinch of citric acid
- Pinch of salt
- Pinch of sugar

For Tempering

- 2 tsp refined oil
- 1/2 tsp mustard seeds
- 1/2 tsp cumin seeds
- 2 tsp sesame seeds
- 2 dry chillies
- Pinch of asafoetida
- 8-10 curry leaves

Preparation

Mix the ingredients for khandvi with 2 cups of water. Put to boil, stirring continuously till thick. To test, spread a little batter on the back of a thali; if it rolls easily the batter is done. If not, cook some more. Then spread the batter quickly on the back side of a large thali evenly and quickly with the help of a spatula. Because this is to be stuffed, do not make the layer thin.

Stuffing: Boil the peas, drain and grind to a paste. Add the remaining ingredients, mix well and remove. Let dry for a minute, then spread the stuffing evenly. Cut into strips and make tight rolls. Heat some oil in a karahi, add the ingredients for the tempering and pour over the Khandvis. Garnish with grated coconut and coriander leaves.

Variation: You may use a pressure cooker for cooking the batter. In that case use 1/2 cup less water and cook for 3 whistles. Mix well and proceed with the recipe.

Instant Dhokla

Ingredients (Serves 2)

- 1/2 cup gramflour
- 1 tbsp semolina
- 1/4 tsp citric acid
- 3/4 tsp Eno's fruit salt
- 1/2 tsp salt

Grind together

- 1/4 cup shelled peas, boiled
- 1 green chilli
- A small piece of ginger

For Tempering

- 1 tbsp refined oil
- 1 tsp sesame seeds
- 1 tsp mustard seeds
- A pinch of asafoetida

Preparation

Mix the gramflour, semolina, citric acid, ground paste and salt together. Add enough water to make a batter of pouring consistency. Lastly add the Eno's fruit salt. Grease a plate and pour in the batter. Steam in a preheated dhokla steamer or pressure cooker for 15-20 minutes. In case you're using a pressure cooker, do not put on the weight. Remove and let cool for half an hour.

Tadka: Heat the oil, temper with the asafoetida, sesame seeds and mustard seeds. Once they pop up, add 1/2 cup of water. Sprinkle the whole thing on the dhokla. Cut and serve.

Variation: Instead of water. add tomato juice to the semolina.

Moong Dal Snack

Ingredients (Serves 4)

- 1 cup moong dal
- 1 small potato, diced
- 1 tbsp refined oil
- 1 tsp roasted and powdered cumin seed
- 1/2 tsp salt
- Pinch of chilli powder
- Lime juice to taste
- 4 slit green chillies for garnishing

Preparation

Soak the dal for an hour. Boil in plenty of water with the potatoes till just done. Do not overcook. Strain. Heat the oil in a non-stick karahi. Add the dal and fry, stirring well, till dry. Sprinkle roasted and powdered cumin, salt, chilli powder and mix well. Serve sprinkled with lime juice to taste and garnished with green chillies.

It is a filling snack, that does not sit heavy in the stomach.

Cabbage Muthia

Ingredients (Serves 4-6)

- 1 cup heaped grated cabbage
- 1 cup heaped gramflour
- 1/2 cup heaped atta
- 1/2 cup grated carrot
- 1/4 tsp bicarbonate of soda
- 1/2 tsp garam masala powder
- 1 tsp salt
- 1 tbsp lime juice
- 1/4 tsp turmeric powder
- Pinch of chilli powder
- Pinch ofasafoetida
- 2 tsp oil

For Tempering

- 1 tsp oil
- 1 tsp urad dal
- 1 tsp mustard seeds
- 10-15 curry leaves
- 1 green chilli, chopped
- A handful of coriander leaves.

Preparation

Muthia: Sieve together the gramflour, atta and soda. Mix all the ingredients and knead to a soft dough. If necessary add a few drops of water. Divide the mixture into 3 sausage shapes. Steam in a pressure cooker for 25 minutes. Open cooker after 5 minutes. The muthias will gain in size and crack at a few places on top. Cut into pieces.

Tempering: Heat the oil in a karahi. Add the urad dal. When it turns darker, add the mustard seeds, then add the green chillies and curry leaves. Stir fry and add the muthias. Fry gently over a medium heat for 2 minutes. Serve with green chutney.

Variation: May use 1 $^{1}/_{2}$ heaped grated bottle gourd the same way.

Gujarati food is very healthy because it relies a lot on steaming. Uses very little oil, too. This muthia is full of fibre and nutrition.

Vegetable Cutlets with Nachni

Ingredients (Makes 12 Cutlets)

- 4 cm piece of ginger
- 5 cloves of garlic
- 1 bunch coriander leaves
- 2 green chillies
- 6 large florets of cauliflower
- 2 medium carrots
- 1 cup shelled green peas
- 3 large potatoes
- 1 large onion
- 100 gm nachni satva
- 3/4 tsp salt
- Semolina as needed
- Refined oil for frying

Preparation

Grind the ginger, garlic, coriander leaves and green chillies to a paste. Cut cauliflower and carrot in small pieces. Finely chop onion. Boil the cauliflower, carrot and peas together till done. Mash coarsely. Separately pressure cook the potatoes with the peel till done, approximately 5-7 minutes. Peel and wash well. Mix the vegetables, potatoes, nachni satva, ground paste, onion and salt. Mix well and knead to a dough without adding water. Take a cellophane or butter paper and sprinkle semolina on it. Take a large lime sized ball of the dough and flatten it over the semolina, sprinkle a little semolina on top. Heat a little oil in a non-stick tava and fry the cutlets on both the sides till golden. Serve hot with a chutney.

Nachni, widely known as ragi, mahua, marua, bawto, ragulu has a high percentage of calcium, higher than in any cereal. The percentage of iodine in it is also the highest.

Masala Roti

Ingredients (Serves 4)

- 6 slices bread
- 1 tbsp refined oil
- 2 tomatoes, chopped
- 1/2 tsp cumin powder
- 1/2 tsp coriander powder
- 1/4 tsp turmeric
- 1/4 tsp chilli powder
- salt to taste

Grind together

- 1 medium onion
- 1 cm ginger
- 2 green chillies
- 6 cloves of garlic
- A handful of coriander leaves

Preparation

Stale breads or even the crusts may be used. Break the breads into coarse pieces and reserve. Heat the oil in a non-stick karahi and add the ground paste. Fry for 5 minutes. Add the tomatoes, spices and salt. Cook. Stir well till the tomatoes are soft and well mixed. Add 1/2 cup of hot water and the bread pieces. Stir to combine well and cook for a few minutes more. Serve hot garnished with fresh coriander. Chappatis and roasted papad will complete the meal.

Bejar Roti

Ingredients (Makes 5-6 Rotis)

- 1/2 cup atta
- 1/2 cup jowar ka atta
- 1/4 cup gramflour
- 1/2 tsp salt
- 1/4 tsp cumin seeds
- 1 tsp green chilli paste
- 2 tbsp chopped mint or fresh coriander

Preparation

Sift the 3 flours and salt. Add rest of the ingredients and knead to a dough with lukewarm water. Keep covered for 30 minutes. Knead well again and divide into small balls. Roll out and bake on a hot tawa till brown spots appear.

Sabji Roti

Ingredients (Serves 2-3)

- 1 cup spinach
- 1/2 cup fenugreek leaves
- 1/4 cup shelled peas
- 1/2 cup french beans
- 1/4 cup coriander leaves
- 1 tsp refined oil
- 1/4 tsp ajwain
- 1 small green chilli
- 1/2 tsp ginger paste
- 1/2 tsp salt
- 250 gm atta

Preparation

Finely chop all the leafy vegetables, beans and green chilli. Steam spinach, fenugreek, peas, beans and coriander leaves without water. Press over a strainer and strain the water. Reserve water. Heat the oil in a non-stick karahi. Add the ajwain and ginger paste. Stir and add the vegetables and saute till dry. You may add a little roasted and powdered cumin and amchur at this stage.

Knead the atta-like chappati dough using the reserved vegetable water. Divide into balls slightly larger than ordinary chappatis. Roll into a circle the size of a puri. Stuff vegetables and shape into a ball again. Roll into a chappati carefully so that the filling does not spill. Put on a tawa on a medium heat and roast till brown spots appear on both the sides.

MISSIE BREAD

Ingredients (Makes one Loaf)

- 1 cup mixed herbs
- 10 gm fresh yeast
- 1 cup milk
- 1 tsp sugar
- 3/4 cup atta
- 3/4 cup jowar ka atta
- 1/2 cup besan
- 1 tsp salt
- 1 tbsp refined oil
- 1 tsp cumin seeds
- 1/2 tsp pepper

Preparation

By mixed herbs I mean coriander leaves, mint, parsley, fenugreek and spinach. Use as many as you can lay your hands on. Crumble the yeast. Dissolve in 1/4 cup lukewarm milk and sugar and leave for 10 minutes. Sift all the flours and salt together. Rub in the oil. Make a bay in the centre of the flour and add the yeast mixture, the remaining milk and the powdered spices. Knead to a soft and pliable dough. Cover and set in a warm place. When it doubles in size, say after 45 minutes to 1 hour, knock back and add the herbs; knead again. Grease a loaf tin and shape the dough in it. Cover and keep for another 20 minutes. It will rise again. Bake in an oven preheated to 180°C/350°F for about 20 minutes. The bread is done when it sounds hollow if tapped with the knuckles.

This homemade bread made with three types of flours is way above in nutrition and taste than any bought variety.

SPINACH AND CHEESE MUFFINS

Ingredients (Makes 12 Muffins)

- 250 gm finely chopped spinach
- 1 cup atta
- 1 cup refined flour
- 1/2 cup wheat bran
- 1 tbsp baking powder
- 1/2 tsp nutmeg powder
- 1 cup grated cheese
- 60 gm paneer, grated
- 1 cup milk
- 1 egg
- 1 tbsp sesame seeds
- Pinch of pepper

Preparation

Remove stalks and any wilted leaves and chop spinach finely. This should weight 250 gm. Steam briefly until just wilted. Cool and squeeze out all moisture. Sift the atta, flour, wheat bran, baking powder, nutmeg and pepper together. Add the cheese and paneer and stir to combine. Beat the egg and combine with the milk. Make a bay in the centre of the flour and add the egg mixture all at once, then add the spinach. Mix the dough lightly. The ingredients should be just combined and the batter should be quite lumpy. Do not over mix. Lightly grease a muffin tray and spoon batter evenly into the holes. Sprinkle with the sesame seeds. Bake in an oven preheated to 190°C/ 360° F for about 25-30 minutes or until nice and golden.

Even those who don't like spinach will fall for this one.

Oat Corn Muffins

Ingredients (Makes 12 Muffins)

- 1/2 cup atta
- 1/2 cup oat bran
- 1/4 tsp salt
- 1 tbsp baking powder
- 1 cup makki ka atta
- Pinch of powdered sugar
- 1 egg
- 2/3 cup milk
- 1/4 tsp green capsico sauce
- 1/4 cup refined oil
- 1/2 capsicum, finely chopped
- 425 g corn kernels
- 1/4 cup fresh coriander, chopped

Preparation

Lightly brush muffins trays with oil. Muffin trays are special ones with holes in them; easily available in the market. You may used tinned corn or fresh ones. Pressure cook fresh ones till soft. Sift the atta, oat bran, salt, baking powder, makki ka atta and sugar together. Combine the egg, milk, capsico and oil in a separate bowl. Make a bay in the centre of the atta mixture. Add the egg mixture, corn, capsicum and coriander all at once. Mix the ingredients until just moisture. Do not overbeat; the batter should be quite lumpy. Because the more you stir, the more gluten develops and tougher the muffin becomes. Spoon the batter evenly into the prepared tin. Bake in an oven preheated to 190°C for 30 minutes. Check after 20 minutes, the tops should be nice and brown and a knife inserted in the middle of the muffin should come out clean.

Try to make bran a part of your daily diet. The following is a modified version of a standard muffin recipe Oat bran is available in health food stores.

Desserts

Lime and Ginger Mousse

Ingredients (Serves 2)

- 100 gm paneer
- 50 gm hung curd
- finely grated rind
- Juice of 1 lime
- 2 tsp gelatine
- Sugar free sweetener equivalent of 2 tbsp sugar
- 1 tsp finely chopped candied ginger
- Slices of lime to decorate

Preparation

Blend paneer and curd till smooth. Place the lime juice in a bowl and sprinkle the gelatine over it. Leave for 5 minutes to 'sponge', then heat over a pan of hot water to dissolve. Allow to cool a little, then stir in all the remaining ingredients and divide between 2 serving glasses. Chill 1 hour or till serving time. Serve decorated with lime slices.

Melon and Strawberry Salad

Ingredients (Serves 4)

- 1 honeydew melon (Kharbuja)
- 12 strawberries
- 150 ml apple juice

Preparation

Peel, halve and deseed the melon. Cut the flesh into bite-sized pieces. Hull the strawberries and halve. Place the melon and strawberries in a large bowl with the apple juice. Toss the fruit and juice well together. Divide between 4 bowls. Chill half an hour and serve.

It is an ideal dessert for a diabetic.

Chocolate Jelly

Ingredients (Serves 2)

- 2 tbsp cocoa powder
- Sugar free sweetener equivalent of 2 tbsp sugar
- 1/4 tsp vanilla essence
- 800 ml skimmed milk
- 2 tsp powdered gelatine
- 2 tsp hung curd

Preparation

Mix together the cocoa powder, sugar free sweetener, vanilla and 3 tbsp of the milk in a small pan till well mixed. Stir in the remaining milk. Bring to the boil and remove from the heat. Sprinkle the gelatine and whisk to dissolve. Divide between 2 dessert bowls and chill to set. Drizzle with 1 tsp of the curd and serve.

The tart flavour of the curd compliments the chocolate beautifully.

Gajrela

Ingredients (Serves 4)

- 2 large carrots
- 500 ml skimmed milk
- Sugar free sweetener to taste

Preparation

Peel and grate the carrots. Cook carrots and milk in a non-stick saucepan till the carrots are soft and the milk reduced. Remove from heat and add the sweetener. Serve hot or cold as desired.

FRUITY FLAVOUR

Ingredients (Serves 4)

- 1 small red apple
- 1 small green apple
- 1 small guava
- 1 orange
- 2 cubes cheese

Dressing

- 1/2 cup hung curd
- 2 tsp chaat masala
- 2 tbsp orange juice
- 1/2 tsp curry powder
- 1/2 tsp grated orange rind
- Pinch of salt
- Pepper to taste

Preparation

Core and dice the apples, but do not peel. Discard the seeds and dice the guava. Segment the orange. Cut the cheese in small dices. Place the fruits decoratively in a serving bowl. Mix the dressing ingredients together. Refrigerate both the fruits and dressing separately. Pour the dressing over the fruits before serving.

Fruits supply carbohydrates and are also a good source of vitamin C. This fruitful dish can be served either as a salad or a dessert.

ANNEXURE

Various Constituents of Food*

Protein, Fat, Carbohydrate and Fibre Content of Foods
(Per 100 gms edible portion)

Food 1	Protein (gm) 2	Fat (gm) 3	Carb (gm) 4	Fibre (gm) 5
Dairy Foods				
Milk whole (Buffalo)	4.3	8.8	5.0	—
Milk whole (Cow)	3.2	4.0	4.4	—
Milk (Skimmed)	2.3	traces	5.0	—
Butter milk	0.8	1.1	0.5	—
Curds	3.1	4.0	3.0	—
Cheese	24.0	25.0	6.0	—
Butter	—	81.0	—	—
Fats and Cooking oils				
Ghee (Cow)	—	100	—	—
Ghee (Buffalo)	—	100	—	—
Hydrogenated cooking oil	—	100	—	—
Groundnut, corn, coconut, mustard	—	100	—	—
Salad Dressings				
Mayonnaise	trace	80	trace	—
French	trace	40	13.3	—
Meat and Poultry foods				
Mutton	18-19	13	0	0
Chicken	18	10	0	0
Duck	21.6	4.8	0.1	0
Beef	22.6	2.6	0	0

*WHO Release, 1986

Contd...

1	2	3	4	5
Pork	19	4.4	—	—
Egg (Hen)	13.3	13.3	—	—
Kidney (Sheep)	21.0	4	—	—
Liver (Sheep)	19.3	8	1.3	—
Ham (Cooked)	24	33	0	0
Fish & Sea-Foods				
Bhetki	14	1	2	—
Pomfret	17	1.3	2	—
Black Pomfret *(Halwa)*	20.3	1.3	2	—
Salmon (Canned)	17	5	0	0
Rohu	17	1.4	4.4	—
Tuna	24	21	0	—
Prawns	21	trace	0	—
Shrimps	17	trace	3	—
Ravas	22.2	1.1	3.3	—
Sardines	21	2	0	—
Mackarels	19	2	0	—
Lobster	21	1	0	—
Sole	16.2	2.3	2.2	—
Pulses and Legumes				
Green gram *(Moong)*	24	1.3	57	4.1
Green gram dal *(Moong dal)*	24.5	1.2	60	0.8
Black gram *(Urad dal)*	24	1.4	60	0.9
Bengal gram dal *(Chana dal)*	21	5.6	60	1.2
Lentil *(Masoor dal)*	25.1	0.7	59	0.7

Contd...

1	2	3	4	5
Red Gram *(Tur Dal)*	22.3	1.7	58	1.5
Rajmah Beans	23	1.3	61	—
Soya beans	43.2	19.5	21	3.7
Vegetables				
Cabbage	2	trace	5	1
Cauliflower	2.6	0.4	4	1.2
Carrots	1	0.2	10.6	1.2
Coriander leaves	3.3	0.6	6.3	1.2
Cucumber	0.4	0.1	2.5	0.4
Brinjals	1.4	0.3	4	1.3
Bittergourd	1.6	0.2	4.2	0.8
Drumstick	2.5	0.1	3.7	5
Lady's Finger *(Bhindi)*	2	0.2	6.4	1.2
Leeks	1.8	0.1	17.2	1.3
Lettuce leaves	2.1	0.3	2.5	0.5
Mint *(Pudina)*	4.8	0.6	6	2
Fenugreek leaves *(Methi Ka Sag)*	4.4	0.9	6	1.1
French-beans	1.7	0.1	4.5	1.8
Beetroot	1.7	0.1	8.8	1
Onions (Small)	1.8	0.1	12.6	0.6
Green Peas (Fresh)	7.2	0.1	16	4
Potatoes *(Alu)*	1.6	0.1	22.6	0.4
Sweet Potatoes	1.2	0.3	28.2	0.8
Radish *(Muli)*				
Spinach *(Palak)*	2	0.7	3.0	0.6
Tomatoes (Fresh)	1	0.2	3.6	0.8
Tomato juice	0.8	trace	4.1	0.25
Tomato (Ketchup)	trace	trace	23.5	trace

Contd...

1	2	3	4	5
Fruits	0.2	0.5	13.4	1.0
Apples	1	0.3	11.6	1
Bananas (Ripe)	1.2	0.3	27.2	0.4
Bananas (Green)	1	1	28	—
Cherries (Red)	1	0.5	13.8	0.4
Coconut (Tender)	1	1	6	—
Currants (Black)	2.7	0.5	75.2	1
Dates (Fresh)	1.2	0.4	34.0	4
Figs	1.3	0.2	7.6	2.2
Grapes (Green variety)	0.5	0.3	16.5	3
Guava (Country)	1	0.3	11.2	5.2
Jackfruit	2	0.3	20	1
Lemon (Sour lime)	1	1	8	2
Lemon (Sweet)	0.7	0.3	7.3	0.7
Lichees	1.4	0.3	14	0.2
Mango (Ripe)	0.6	0.4	16.9	0.7
Melon (Water)	0.2	0.2	3.3	0.2
Orange	0.7	0.2	10.9	0.2
Orange (Juice)	0.2	0.1	2	—
Peaches	1.2	0.3	10.5	1.2
Papaya (Ripe)	0.6	0.1	7.2	0.8
Pears	0.6	0.2	11.9	1.0
Pineapple	0.4	0.1	10.8	0.5
Plums (Red)	0.7	0.5	11.1	0.4
Pomegranate	1.6	0.1	14.5	5.1
Raisin (Kishmish)	1.8	0.3	74.6	1.1
Seetaphal (Custard apple)	1.6	0.4	23.5	3.1
Sapota *(Chiku)*	0.7	1.1	21.4	2.6
Strawberries	0.7	0.2	10	1.1
Sugar-cane	trace	0	20	3
Sugar-cane juice	trace	0	20	3

Contd...

1	2	3	4	5
Cereal and Cereal foods				
Bajra	11.6	5	68	1
Barley	11.5	1.3	19.6	4
Jowar	10.4	2	72.6	1.6
Oatmeal	13.6	7.6	63	3.5
Rice raw (Milled)	7	0.5	78.2	0.2
Rice raw (Unmilled)	7.5	1.0	76.7	0.6
Vermicelli	9	trace	78	trace
Wheat flour				
Wheat *(Atta)*	12.1	1.7	69.4	2
Wheat flour				
(refined) *(Maida)*	11	1	74	0.3
Bread (White)	7.8	0.7	52	0.2
Wheat germ	29.2	7.4	53.3	1.4
Bread (Brown)	9	1.4	49.50	1.2
Biscuits (Sweet)	6.4	15.2	72	—
Biscuits (Salted)	6.6	32.4	54.6	—
Nuts and Seeds				
Almonds	21	59	11	2
Cashewnuts	21	47	22	1
Coconut (Dried)	7	62	18	7
Groundnuts	32	40	19	3
(Roasted)				
Pistachio nuts	20	54	16	2
Walnuts	16	65	11	3
Miscellaneous				
Arrowroot flour	0	0	83	—
Cocoa powder	20	25	30	—
Honey	0.3	0	79.5	—
Jaggery (Date palm)	1.5	0.3	86.1	—
Sago	0.2	0.2	87.1	—
Papads	19	0.3	52.4	—

Contd...

1	2	3	4	5
Jam	0	0	70	—
Milk Chocolate	3.6	10.7	79	trace
Coffee (Normal)	trace	5	5	—
Tea (Leaves)	8	4	70	6
	Protein	Fat	Carb	% Alc.
Carbonated drinks (Artificially sweetened)	0	0	0	—
Carbonated soda	0	0	0	—
Cola drinks (Sweetened)	0	0	11	—

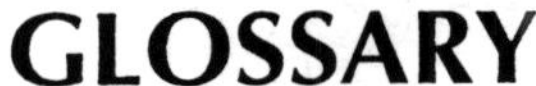

GLOSSARY

FOODGRAINS

English	Spiked millet	Barley	Jowar	Italian millet	Maize (dry)	Oatmeal	Ragi
Hindi	Bajra	Jau	Juar-janera	Kangri	Makai	Jai	Okra
Tamil	Cambu	Barli arisi	Cholam	Thenai	Muka cholam	—	Ragi
Telugu	Gantelu	Barli biyyam	Jonnalu	Korralu	Mekka jonnalu	—	Chollu
Marathi	Bajri	Juv	Jwari	Rala	Muka	—	Nachni
Bengali	Bajra	Job	Juar	Syamadhan kangni	Sukna paka bhutta	Jai	—
Gujarati	Bajri	Jau	Juar	Ral kang	Makai	—	Ragi bhav
Malayalam	Kamboo	Yavam	Cholam	Thina	Unakku cholam	Oat mavu	Moothari (korra)
Kannada	—	—	Jola	—	Vonugida musikinu	Jolu	Ragi
Kashmiri	Baajr'u	Wushku	—	Shol	Makka'y	—	—

Contd...

Foodstuff	Rice (raw)	Rice (parboiled)	Rice (white)	Rice (black)	Rice flakes	Rice (puffed)	Samai
Hindi	Arwa chawal	Usna chawal	Safed chaval	Chaval (kala)	Chowla	Murmura	Kutki, Sanwali
Tamil	Pachai arisi	Puzhungal arisi	Vellai puttu arisi	Karuppu puttu arisi	Arisi aval	Arisia pori	Samai
Telugu	Pachi biyyam	Uppudu biyyam	Thella biyyam	Nalla biyyam	Atukulu	Murmuralu	—
Marathi	Tandool	Tandool ukda	—	—	Pohe	Murmure	Sava
Bengali	Atap chowl	Siddha chowl	—	—	Chaler khood	Muri	Kangni
Gujarati	Hatna	Ukadelloo chokha	—	—	Pohva	Mumra	—
Malayalam	Pacchari	Puzhungal ari	Velutha puttari	Karutha puttari	Avil	Pori	—
Kannada	Kotnuda	Kotnuda	—	—	Avalukki	—	Puri
Kashmiri	—	—	—	—	—	—	—

Contd...

English	Semolina	Vermicelli	Wheat (whole)	Wheat flour (whole)	Wheat flour (refined)	Wheat (broken)
Hindi	Sooji	Siwain	Gehun	Atta	Maida	Daliya
Tamil	Ravai	Semiya	Godumai	Muzhu godmai ma	Maida mavu	Godhumbi ravai
Telugu	Rawa	Semiya	Godhumalu	Godhum pindi	Maidha pindi	Dinchina gadhumalu
Marathi	—	Shevaya	Gahu	Gahu kuneek	Gahu kuneek	Gavache satva
Bengali	Suji	Sewai	Gomasta	Atta	Maida	Bhanga gom
Gujarati	—	—	Ghau	Ato	—	Fadia ghaun
Malayalam	Rava	Semiya	Muzhu gothambu	Gothambu mavu	Maidu tha gothambu mavu	Gothumbu ari
Kannada	—	Shavige	Godhi	Godhi	Hittu madia	Kuttida Godhi
Kashmiri	—	Ku' nu'	—	—	—	—

VEGETABLES

English	Ash gourd	Bitter gourd	Bottle gourd	Brinjal	Broad beans	Cabbage	Capsicum
Hindi	Safed petha	Karela	Ghia	Baingan	Sem	Bandhgobi	Simla mirch
Bengali	Chal kumdo	karala	Laoo	Begoon	Sheem	Badha kopee	Lonka
Assamese	Lao bishesh	—	Jati lao	Bengena	Urahi	Bondhakobi	Kashmiri jalakai
Oriya	Pani kakkaru	—	Lau	Baigana	Shimba	Patrokobi	Simla lonka
Marathi	Kohala	Karle	Dudhi	Wangi	Ghewda	Pan kobi	Bhopli mirchi
Gujarati	Petha	Karela	Dudhi	Ringna	Papdi	Kobi	Simla marchan
Telugu	Boodie gumadi	Kakara	Sorakaya	Vankaya	Pedda chikkudu	Kosu	Pedda mirappa
Kannada	Budu gumbala	Hagalkai	Sorekai	Badanekai	Chapparadavare	Kosu	Donne menasinakai
Tamil	Pooshanikkai	Pavakkai	Suraikai	Kaththarikai	Avaraikai	Muttaikosu	Kuda milakai
Malayalam	Kumbalanga	Kaypakka	Cheraikai	Vazhutheninga	Amarakai	Muttakose	Parangi mulagu
Kashmiri	Masha'ly al	Karelu	—	Waangun	—	Bandgobhi	—

Contd...

English	Carrot	Cauliflower	Cluster beans	Colocasia	Coriander leaves	Cucumber	Curry leaves
Hindi	Gajar	Phulgobi	Guar ki phalli	Arvi	Hara Dhania	Khira	Kadi patta
Bengali	Gujar	Foolcopy	Jhar sim	—	Dhonay pata	Sasha	Curry pata
Assamese	Gajor	Phoolkobi	—	Kochu	Dhania paat	—	Narasingha paat
Oriya	Gajar	Phulakobi	—	—	Dhania patra	—	Bhrusanga patta
Marathi	Gajar	Fulkobi	Govari	Alu kanda	Kothimbir	Kakari	Kadhi patta
Gujarati	Gajar	Fool kobi	Govar	Alvi	Kothmir	Kakdi	Mitho limdo
Telugu	Gajjara	Cauliflower	Goruchikkudu kayalu	Chamadumpa	Kothimeera	Dosakaya	Karivepaku
Kannada	Gajjari	Hookosu	Gorikayi	Keshave	Kottambari soppu	Southaikayi	Karibevu
Tamil	Carrot	Koveppu	Kothavarangai	Seppann kizhangu	Koththamali ilaigal	Kakkarikkai	Kariveppilai
Malayalam	Carrot	Coliflower	Kothavara	Chembu	Kothamalli ila	Vellari	Kariveppila
Kashmiri	—	Phoolgobhi	—	—	—	Laa'r	—

Contd...

English	Drumstick	French beans	Garlic	Ginger (fresh)	Green chillies	Jackfruit	Lady's finger
Hindi	Sahjan ki phali	Pharsbeen	Lassan	Adrak	Hari mirch	Kathal	Bhindi
Bengali	Sajane dauta	French beans	Rasoon	Ada (tatka)	Kancha lonka	Echore	Dhanroce
Assamese	Sajina	Faras been	Naharoo	Ada (kesa)	Kesa jalakia	—	Bhendi
Oriya	Sajana chhuin	French beans	Rasuna	Ada (kancha)	Kancha lonka	—	Bhendi
Marathi	Shevgyachya shenga	Farasbi	Lasun	Aale	Hirvya mirchya	Kawla phanas	Bhendi
Gujarati	Saragvani shing	Fansi	Lasan	Adu	Lila marcha	Phunas	Bhinda
Telugu	Munagakayalu	French chikkudu	Vellulli	Allam (pachchi)	Pachchi mirapakayalu	Letha panasa	Bendakaaya
Kannada	Nuggekai	Avare	Bellulli	Ashi Shunti	Hasi menasinakai	Yele halasu	Bendekai
Tamil	Murungaikai	Beans	Ulli Poondu	Inji	Pachchai milagai	Pila pinchu	Vendaikai
Malayalam	Muringakkaya	Beans	Veluthulli	Inji	Pachamulagu	Idichakka	Vendakka
Kashmiri	—	—	Ruhan	—	Myool martsu waungun	—	Bindu

Contd...

English	Lettuce	Lemon	Mint leaves	Onion	Parwal	Peas	Plantain flower	Plantain green
Hindi	Salad ke patte	Nimbu	Pudina	Pyaz	Parwal	Matar	Kele ka phool	Kacha kela
Bengali	Lettuce	Lebu	Poodina pata	Pyaz	Potol	Motor	Mocha	Kancha kala
Assamese	Laipaat	Nemu	Podina	—	Patol	Motormah	—	—
Oriya	Lettuce	Lembu	Podana patra	—	Potala	Matar	—	—
Marathi	Saladchi paane	Limbu	Pudina	Kanda	—	Matar	Kel phool	Kele
Gujarati	Lettuce	Limbu	Fudino	Dungli	—	Vatana	Kelphool	Kela
Telugu	Lettuce koora	Nimma	Pudhina koora	Nirulli	—	Bathanedu	Aratipuwu	Arati kayi
Kannada	Lettuce soppu	Nimbu	Pudina sopu	Erulli	—	Betani	Balo mothu	Bala kayi
Tamil	Lettuce keerai	Elumicham pazham	Pudhinaa	Vengayam	—	Pattani	Vazhaippu	Vazhaikkai
Malayalam	Uvarcheera	Cherunaranga	Pudhinaa	Ulli	—	Pattani Payaru	Vazhappoo	Vazhakka
Kashmiri	Salaad	—	—	Gandu	—	Matar	—	—

Contd...

English	Plantain stem	Potato	Radish	Red pumpkin	Ridge gourd	Snake gourd	Sweet potato	Yam elephant
Hindi	Kele ka tana	Aloo	Muli	Sitaphal	Torai	—	Shakarkand	Zaminkand
Bengali	Thor	Aloo	Mulo	Ronga Koomra	Jhinge	Chichinga	Rangalu	Kham aloo
Assamese	—	Alu	—	Ronga lao	—	—	—	Kaath aloo
Oriya	—	Alu	—	Kakharu	—	—	—	Deshi alu
Marathi	Kelecha khunt	Batate	Mula	Lal bhopla	Dodka	Pudwal	Ratale	Suran
Gujarati	Kelanu thed	Batata	Mula	Kolu	Turai	Pandola	Sakkaria	Suran
Telugu	Arati davva	Bangaala dumpa	Mullangi	Erra gummadi	Beerakai	Potlakayi	Dumpalu	Kanda dumpa
Kannada	Dindu	Aalugadde	Mullangi	Kempu kumbala	Heeraikai	Padavalai	Genasu	Suvarnagadde
Tamil	Vazhaithandu	Urulaikizhangu	Mullangi	Parangikai	Pirrkkankai	Podalangai	Sarkarai valli kizhangu	Chenai kizhangu
Malayalam	Vazhappindi	Uralakkizhangu	Mullangi	Chuvappu mathan	Pecchinga	Padavalanga	Chakkara kizhangu	Chena
Kashmiri	—	Oloo	Muj	Paarimal	Turrelu	—	—	—

PULSES

English	Bengal gram (whole)	Bengal gram (split)	Black gram (split)	Black gram (whole)	Cornflour	Cow gram`	Green gram (whole)
Hindi	Chana	Chana dal	Urad dal	Sabat urad	Makai ka atta	Lobia (bada)	Moong
Bengali	Chola	Banglar chhola	Mashkolair dal	Mashkolai dal	Bhoottar maida	Barbati	Mug
Assamese	—	Buttor dail	Matir dail (phola)	Matir dail (gota)	Moida	—	—
Oriya	—	Buta (chhota)	Biri (phala)	Biri (gota)	Makka atta	—	—
Marathi	Hurbhura	Chana dal	Udid dal	Udid	Makyache pith	Kuleeth	Mug
Gujarati	Chana	Chana nidaal	Adad ni dal	Adad	Makai no lot	—	Mag
Telugu	Sanagalu	Senaga pappu	Mina pappu	Minu mulu	Mokkajonnalu (pindi)	Ada chandalu	Pesalu
Kannada	Kadale	Kadale bela	Uddina bela	Uddu	Musukinajolada hittu	Thadaguni	Hesaru kalu
Tamil	Muzhu kadalai	Kadalai paruppu	Ulutham paruppu	Ulundhu	Chola Maavu	Karamani	Pachai payaru
Malayalam	Kadala	Kadala parippu	Uzhunnu parrippu	Uzhunnu	Cholapodi	Payar	Cherupayaru
Kashmiri	Chanu	—	Maha	—	—	—	Muang

Contd...

English	Green gram (split)	Horse gram	Kesari dal	Kidney beans	Red gram	Red lentils	Soya bean
Hindi	Moong dal	Kulthi	Lang dal	Rajma	Arhar dal	Masoor dal	Bhat
Bengali	Moog	Kulthi kalai	Khesari	Barbati beej	Arhar dal	Lal masoor (bhanga)	Gari kalai
Assamese	Sevjiy Boot	—	—	Markhowa urahi	Rahor dail	Masoor dail (phola)	—
Oriya	Muga (Phala)	—	—	Baragudi chhuin	Harada dali	Masura dali (phala)	—
Marathi	Moog dal	Kuleeth	Lakh dal	—	Tur dal	Masur dal	Soya
Gujarati	Magnidal	Kuleeth	Lakh	—	Tuver dal	Masur dal	Soya
Telugu	Pesaru pappu	Ulavalu	Lamka pappu	—	Kandi pappu	Missu pappu	—
Kannada	Hesare bele	Huruli	—	—	Togar bele	Masur bele	—
Tamil	Pasi paruppu	Kollu	Vattuparuppu	—	Thuvaram parappu	Massor paruppu	—
Malayalam	Cherupayar parippu	Muthira	—	—	Thuvara parippu	Masoor parippu	Soya bean
Kashmiri	—	—	—	—	—	Musur	—

Fruits and Dry Fruits

English	Almond	Coconut	Currants	Dates	Dry plums
Hindi	Badam	Nariyal	Mungaqqa	Khajur	Alu bukhara
Bengali	Badam	Narcole	Manaca	Khejoor	Sookno kool
Assamese	Badam	Narikol	Kismis	Khejur	Sukan bogori
Oriya	Badaam	Nadia	Kala kismis	Khajura	Barakoli jateeya phala
Marathi	Badam	Naral	Manuka	Khajur	Alubhukar
Gujarati	Badam	Naliyer	Kalli draksh	Khajoor	Suka Plum
Telugu	Badam	Kobbari kaaya	Endu nalla dhraksha	Kharjoora pandu	—
Kannada	Badami	Tenginakai	Dweepa dharakshi-kappu	Kharjoora	—
Tamil	Badam/vadhumai	Thengai	Karumdhraakshai	Perichampazham	Aalpacota ular pazham
Malayalam	Badam	Nalikeram/Thenga	Karuthamurthiri	Eethapazham	—

Contd...

English	Guavas	Lemon	Orange	Raisins	Walnuts
Hindi	Amrud	Nimbu	Santra	Kishmish	Akhrot
Bengali	Payara	Lebu	Kamla lebu	Kishmish	Akhrot
Assamese	Madhurium	Nemu	Sumothira	Sukan angoor	Akhrot
Oriya	Pijuli	'Lembu	Kamala	Kismis	Akhrot
Marathi	Peru	Limbu	Santre	Bedane	Akrod
Gujarati	Jamrukh	Limbu	Santara	Lal draksh	Akhrot
Telugu	Jaamapandu	Nimma	Kamala Pandu	Kismis pallu	Aakrot
Kannada	Seebe	Nimbe	Kittale	Dweepadrakshi	Acrota
Tamil	Koyyapazham	Elumicham pazham	Kichilipazham	Ular dhraakshai	Akhrot
Malayalam	Perakkai	Cherunaranga	Madhura naranga	Unakkamunthiri	Akrotandi

Dry Spices

English	Aniseed	Asafoetida	Basil leaves	Bay leaf	Caraway seeds	Cardamom (brown)	Cardamom (green)	Cinnamon
Hindi	Saunf	Hing	Tulse ke patte	Tej patta	Shahjeera	Moti elaichi	Choti elaichi	Dalchini
Bengali	Mowri	Hing	Tulsi pata	Tej pata	Sajeera	Elach (tamate)	Elach (sobooj)	Daroochini
Assamese	Guwamori	Hing	Tulosi paat	Tejpaat	Bilati jira	Ilachi (muga)	Ilachi (sevjia)	Dalcheni
Oriya	Panamahuri	Hengu	Tulasi patra	Teja patra	Sahajira	Aleicha	Gijuratie	Dalachini
Marathi	Badishep	Hing	Tulsichi paney	Tamal patra	Shahjeera	Masala welchi	Welchi (hirvi)	Dalchini
Gujarati	Variyali	Hing	Tulsina pan	Tamal patra	Jiru	Elcho	Lila alchi	Tuj
Telugu	Sopaginja	Inguva	Thulasi akulu	—	Seema sopyginjale	Yalakulu	Yala kulu (pachavi)	Dalchina chekka
Kannada	Sopubeeja	Hingu	Tulasi ele	—	Caraway beejagalre	Yalakki	Yalakki (hasuru)	Dalchini
Tamil	Perumjeerakam	Perungaayam	Thulasi	—	Karunjeerakam	Elakkai (Pazhuppu)	Elakkai (pachchai)	Lavangapattai
Malayalam	Perumjeerakam	Kaayam	Tulasi	—	Karunjeerakam	Elakkaya	Pach Elakkaya	Karuvapatta
Kashmiri	—	Yangu	—	—	—	Aal budu'a aal	—	—

Contd...

English	Cloves	Coriander seeds	Cumin seeds	Fenugreek seeds	Mace	Mustard seeds	Nutmeg	Parsley
Hindi	Laung	Sukha dhania	Jeera	Methi dana	Javitri	Rai	Jaiphal	Ajmooda ka patta
Bengali	Labango	Dhonay	Jeera	Methi	Jaeetri	Sarsay	Jaifall	Parsley
Assamese	Long	Dhania guti	Gota jeera	Paleng	Janee	Sarioh guti	Jaaiphal	Sugandhi lota
Oriya	Labanga	Dhania	Jira	Methi	Jayatree	Sorisha	Jaiphala	Balabalua shaga
Marathi	Lavanga	Dhane	Jire	Methi dane	Jaypatri	Mohari	Jayphal	Ajmoda
Gujarati	Laving	Dhana	Jeeru	Methi	Jaypatra	Rai	Jaypal	Ajmo
Telugu	Lavangalu	Dhaniyalu	Jeelakara	Menthulu	Japathri	Aavaalu	Jaikaaya	Kothimeerajaii koora
Kannada	Lavanga	Kottambari beeja	Jeerige	Menthe	Japatri	Sasive kalu	Jaika	Kottambari jotiya soppu
Tamil	Kraambu	Koththamali virai	Jeerakam	Vendhayam	Jaadipathri	Kadugu	Jaadhikai	Kothamalu ilaigal pole
Malayalam	Karayaamboovu	Kothamalli	Jeerakam	Uluva	Jathipathri	Kadugu	Jathikka	Malliela pole
Kashmiri	Ru'ang	Daaniwal	Zyur	—	Jalwatur	—	Zaaphal	

Contd...

English	Peppercorns	Pomegranate seeds	Poppy seeds	Red Chillies	Tamarind	Turmeric	Vinegar	Thymol
Hindi	Kali mirch ke daane	Anardana	Khus khus	Lal mirch	Imli	Haldi	Sirka	Ajwain
Bengali	Marich	Dareem bij	Posto	Paka lonka	Tentool	Halood	Seerka	—
Assamese	Jaluk	Dalim guti	—	Sukan jalakia	Teteli	Halodhi	Sirika	—
Oriya	Golamaricha	Dalimba manji	—	Nali lankamaricha	Tentuli	Haladi	Vinegar	—
Marathi	Kale Miri	Dalimbache dane	Khas khas	Lal mirchya	Chincha	Halad	Sirka	Onva
Gujarati	Mari	Dadamna bee	Khaskhas	Lal marcha	Amli	Haldar	Sirko	Ajmo
Telugu	Miriyaalu	Daanimma ginjalu	Gasagasaalu	Erra mirapa kayalu	Chinthapandu	Pasupu	—	—
Kannada	Menasina kalu	Dalimbo beeja	Gasagase beeja	Kempu menasinakai	Hunase hannu	Arasina	—	—
Tamil	Milagu	Maadhulai vidhai	Kasakasaa	Milagai vatal	Puli	Manjal	Pulikaadi	—
Malayalam	Kurumulagu	Madhala naranga kuru	Kaskas	Chuvanna Mulagu	Puli	Manjal	Vinagiri	—

More Books on Diet & Nutrition

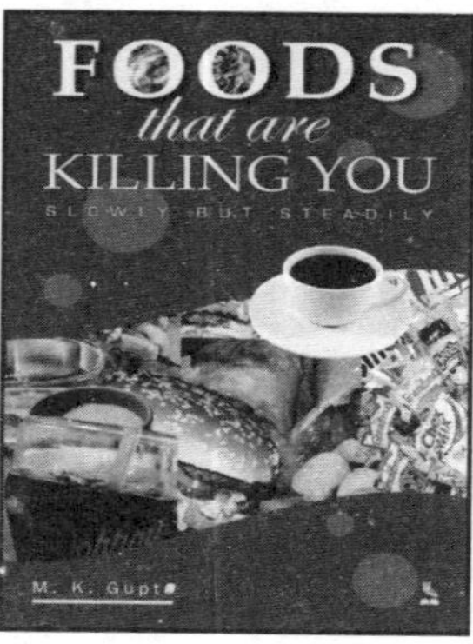

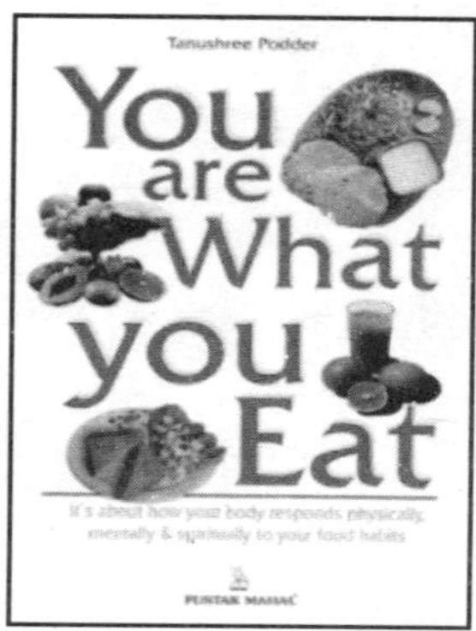

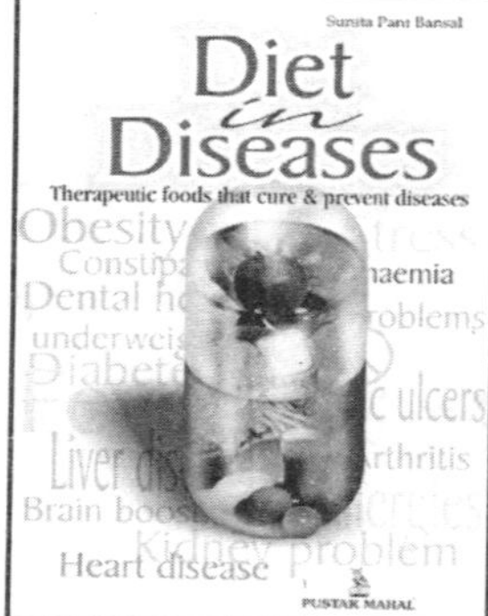

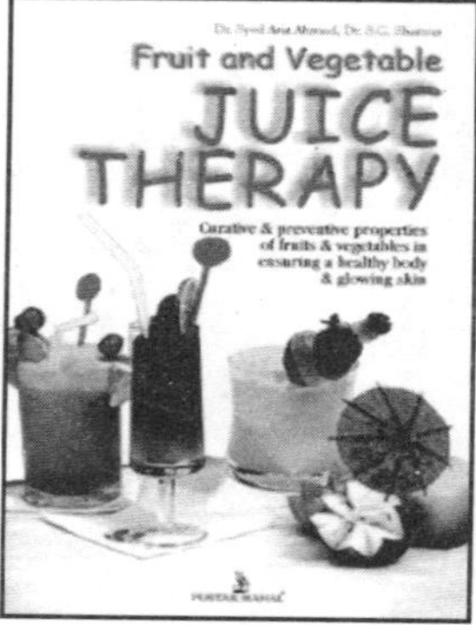

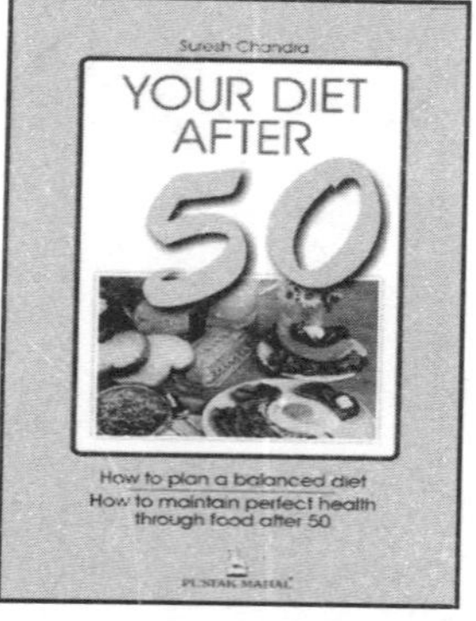

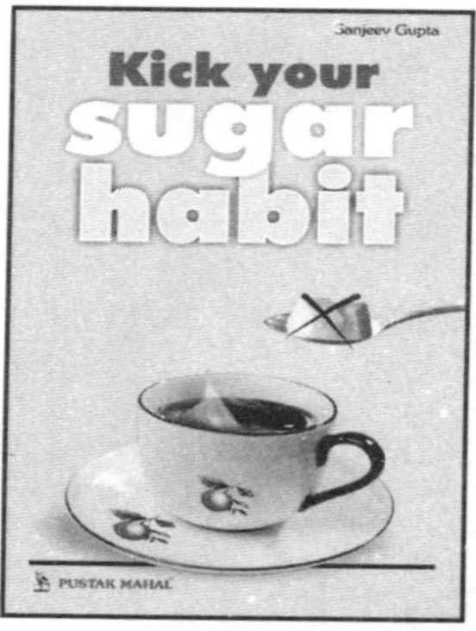

More Books on Health Remedies

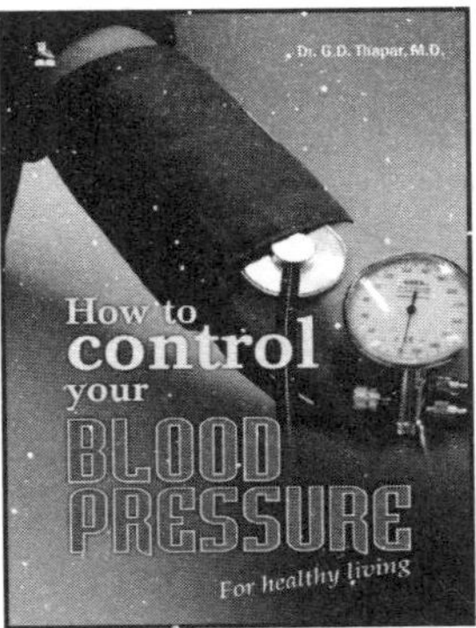

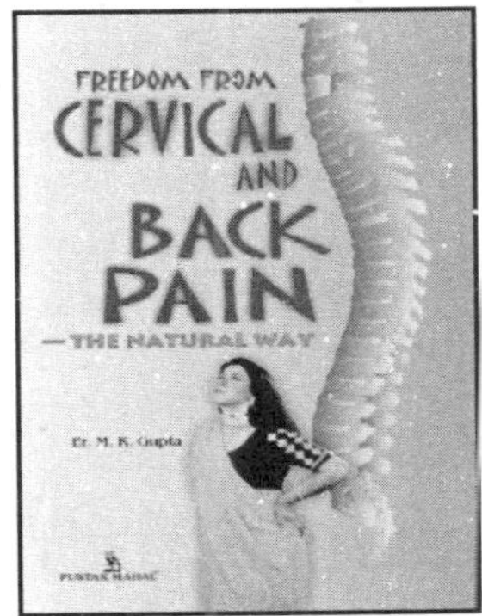

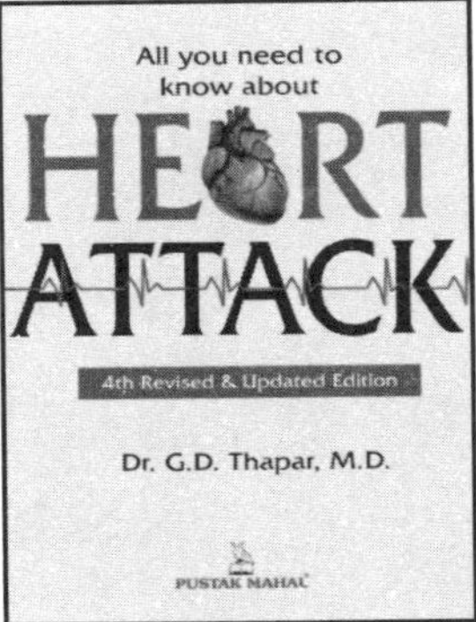

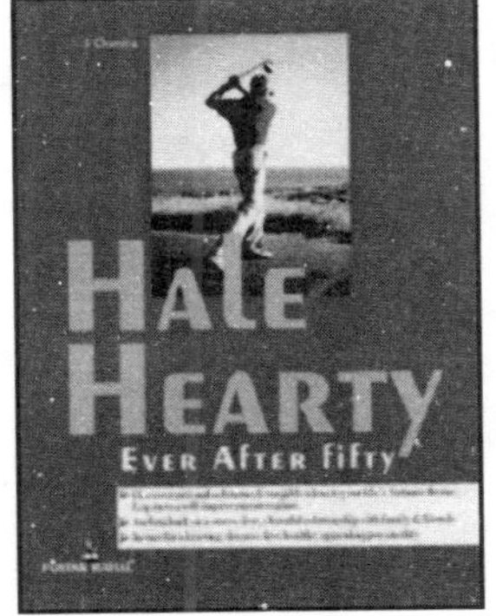

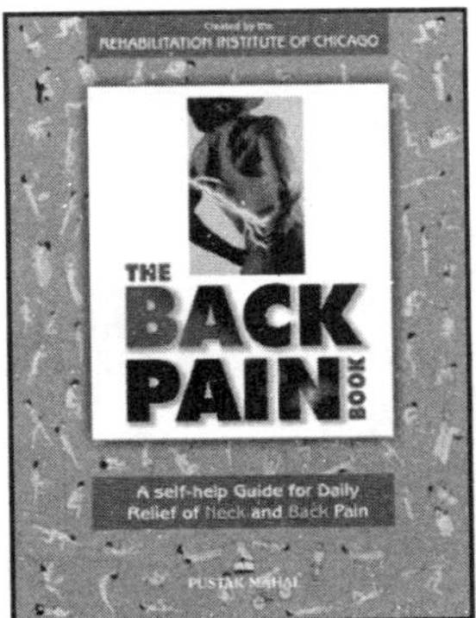

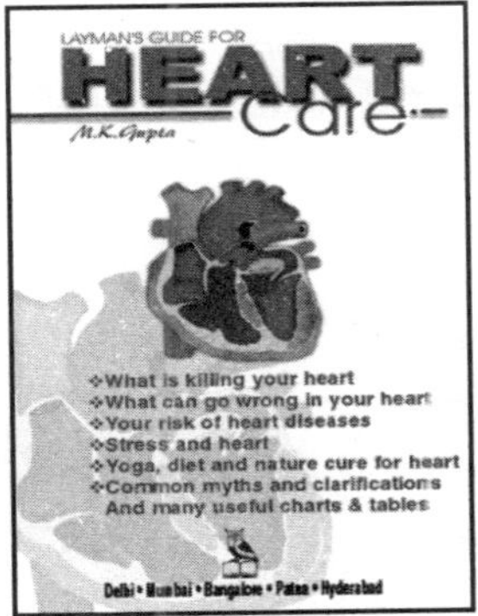